Here's everything that you need to know about marketing in 31 words.

People don't want cheap, they want easy. They want perceived innovation, not slight improvement. And people don't want the best, they want to trust that whatever they are buying isn't crap.

Grab a coffee, or tea, or protein shake. It's time to get going. I'm happy you're here, and ready to make some magic with you. Let's do this!

Welcome to the Wealthy Fit Pro Series

The fitness industry is beautifully flawed. It simultaneously transforms lives and chews up and spits out many of its top change agents. If you want to stick around, you must learn what the certification programs don't teach: the business and marketing necessary for success.

The Wealthy Fit Pro's Guides gather the brightest minds in the global fitness industry to bring you the guidance you need at the lowest price possible. You hold in your hands book three in this series: *Getting Clients and Referrals.* By far the most common question trainers ask me is, "How do I get more clients?" This book is the answer.

I embraced the challenge of this series because when I started my career I felt alone. I was lucky to come across mentors and read the right books at the right time. If we want to make the world a better, healthier place, it starts with passionate fit pros like you. You have the potential to change lives, but it won't happen if you can't make the money that you deserve.

I'm happy you're here and excited for your career. Welcome, and let's dig in!

—Coach Jon

*P.S. This book is the beginning. I'd love to connect with you more. Feel free to friend me on my personal Facebook page at **theptdc.com/fb** and send me a message anytime. My entire team and I are here for you.*

The Wealthy Fit Pro's Guide to Getting Clients and Referrals
ISBN: 9781706797845

Cover and interior book design by Growler Media

Bulk order discounts are available for fitness centers, education companies, academic institutions, and mentorships. Please inquire by emailing support@theptdc.com with subject line "bulk book order."

The Wealthy Fit Pro's Guide to

GETTING CLIENTS AND REFERRALS

JONATHAN GOODMAN

WITH MIKE DOEHLA AND 14 OF THE FITNESS INDUSTRY'S LEADING VOICES

CONTENTS

INTRODUCTION

Why People Pay for Fitness When They Can Get It for Free

Fitness has *always* been free.

It costs nothing to run, jump, and play. Just about anybody can get into shape using free outdoor or community resources available to them.

Anybody with an internet connection can access hundreds of thousands of free workout programs. Same with nutrition guides and recipes.

So why is the global health and fitness industry worth more than a trillion dollars? And why are so many consumers willing to pay a premium for something they really don't need to pay for?

An even better question: How can you add enough value to *your* service so people beg to buy something from you that they can get for free elsewhere?

This book has the answers.

Our journey starts by talking about the most important person in the world — you.

A client walks into a gym ...

Odds are once a client contacts you, they've likely already looked up YouTube videos, perused a few websites, followed a few fitness experts on Facebook, and maybe even bought a book or two.

As a result, he'll have preconceptions of what he believes is the *right* approach to fitness. You may agree with him. You may not.

Point is, if you wait until he walks into the gym to impress upon him the importance of *your* wonderful/special/unprecedented approach to fitness, you're four to six months too late. He'll already believe something and it's going to be hard to change his mind.

The barrier to the fitness market is so low it's barely a speed bump. Anybody can develop a (free) website, upload some (phone) photos, give their (un)educated opinion, and broadcast their (supposed) expertise on social media. Sometimes this information is good. Other times ... not so much.

The first fact you must understand is that the fitness industry has become both democratized and decentralized. Power is no longer held by a central few big players in the space. Any person can enter and broadcast at will. The resulting market effects of this kind of disruption have fundamentally shifted how you must approach the business.

Back when fitness was mostly a local thing, as long as

you happened to be located close to a prospect you had a pretty good chance of both convincing her of your way of training and converting her into a client.

Times have changed. The modern-day industry has been disrupted, creating **infinite shelf space.**

This isn't unique to the fitness industry, of course. Picture your local bookstore with aisles and stacks and tables of books. Even the biggest stores had a finite amount of space in which to stock books. Amazon changed that. Instead of choosing between the books at a bookstore, now you can select from millions of titles from the comfort of your couch. The same has happened with fitness. <u>The resulting effect is not deadening competition but *tremendous opportunity*</u> to those willing to understand it. Which includes you now that you're reading this book. :)

Infinite shelf space has fundamentally changed the way people buy. Two things happen in any decentralized, democratized market:

1. **The cream always rises to the top.** Because the power shifts back to consumers, quality will always win, even if it takes some time.
2. **Only a few win big, but tons win.** Without gatekeepers, a few players will be able to build huge businesses. At the same time, a ton of smaller businesses that otherwise wouldn't have had much opportunity will thrive.

Feel overwhelmed or intimidated? Don't. It's very

good news for you. Most fit pros are still terrible at marketing; they've yet to discover the principles you're about to learn. There's more opportunity for you now than ever before. But to take advantage, you have to be willing to do something most people don't: *You have to open your mind to the power of you.*

For the record, that does *not* mean having the biggest ego or the loudest mouth. It does mean solving that central mystery about why people spend money.

Where you fit in the evolving fitness marketplace

Like I said, the burden of entry to the market is close to zero.

- Certifications are cheap and easy, and online you don't even need one.
- Most trainers operate without insurance.*
- Websites are free and easy to set up.
- You can produce free content with the phone in your pocket and reach anybody in the world through social media.

So let's really get into this: The first stage in a decentralized market? A widening wealth gap. A few win big and many become frustrated. The people who figure out how to trick the tools (and get lucky) take

---

* *I'm not saying that this is a good idea. It is, however, the reality.*

home a vast majority of the riches.

We've been in this first stage for a while. It's discouraged a lot of good fit pros.

Everything, however, swings with the pendulum. When decentralization starts, it knocks the pendulum off kilter and everything gets nutty. Over time, the market regulates itself and things settle.

We're just now entering the more stable stage. The more stable one. Nutty stuff will still happen. This is the fitness industry, after all, and nutty stuff always happens. But once we're firmly in the second stage, we'll stay there for many years because it's much more stable than the current ecosystem. What are the hallmarks of this new stage?

- *The power flows back to the consumer.* Reputational damage* takes out low-quality producers because public review communities become more powerful and accessible. Unhappy clients share details about lousy service and results.

- *Increases in cost-to-market across the board.* Rising ad costs, fractured customer attention, and rapid

---

* Additionally, your reputation becomes your biggest asset and you must protect it at all costs. On the internet, it doesn't matter who's right or wrong in a disagreement. By the time somebody complains, it's too late.

Unfortunately, this also calls for extremely loose refund policies and appeasements to customers even if they're clearly in the wrong — for no other reason than it's cheaper to appease them than it is to have them make anything public. You must include this as a cost of doing business and incorporate it into your cost structure moving forward.

decline of organic reach mean large, previously influential companies and individuals can no longer shelter and monopolize audiences.

- *Smaller service providers will see unprecedented opportunity.* That means *you*, and that's very exciting. A decentralized market is impossible to completely target, which means that the value of playing at the fringes for smaller providers increases.

How to get somebody to choose you (and not consider anybody else)

Back to the mystery: Something happens to make a prospect want a coach, online or in-person, bad enough to seek one out. When they do, they're presented with countless options — infinite shelf space — and unless you give them a reason to believe otherwise, they have no idea how to differentiate.

Choosing is hard. Choosing sucks. Whoever makes the decision as easy as possible for the prospect often gets the sale.

I can't express in words just how exciting this is, so I'll hand it off to Online Trainer Academy Head Coach Alex Cartmill:

> *"The greatest marketing advantage you have, and will always have, is that there is only one of you."*

Most fit pros market themselves based on the 99 percent that makes them the same as everybody else. They help "BURN FAT," or "PACK ON MUSCLE," or "LOSE THE BABY WEIGHT," or whatever.

That way of thinking may be the biggest blind spot for well-intentioned trainers today. *You'll have a difficult time marketing thinner, faster, stronger, or lighter because your audience has seen it all before, been promised it all, and tried it all.* As a result, they don't believe you, and, more important, **they don't believe in themselves**.

If you were the first person to market "lose fat and gain muscle," you'd be golden. But you're not the first, second, third, or in the top few thousand. Odds are any potential client you speak to has tried and failed to make the very transformation that you're promising to help him with.

The trainers who have prospects lining up, asking to buy, have found new paths. Heed the words of legendary advertiser Eugene Schwartz:

> *"If your market is at the stage where they've heard all the claims, in all their extremes, then mere repetition or exaggeration won't work any longer. What this market needs now is a new device to make all these claims become fresh and believable to making them again. In other words, A NEW MECHANISM — a new way to making the old promise work. A different process — a fresh chance — a brand-new possibility of success*

where only disappointment has resulted before."

Imagine going to a store to buy a TV and each one has a sign on it saying, "We show you a moving picture." Sure, all you want is a moving picture. But you could never admit that. And, even if you could, how would you ever decide? *Every single TV has a moving picture.* If this happened, the paradox of choice would be paralyzing.

The majority of fitness consumers are not educated in what makes a great trainer or even in what they really need. As a result, purchasing the services of a fitness professional is almost never a merit-based decision simply because it would be too difficult for the average Joe or Jane to analyze who or what is better.

Despite this, most fit pros still tend to market themselves based on the equivalent of the television analogy — they help burn fat, gain muscle, lose the baby weight, whatever. The result: For most consumers, making a decision becomes so difficult that it either never happens, or they make a bad decision because it's easier.

This sucks. We must do better.

Gathering appropriate info to make a purchase decision is difficult. And tedious. And humans like me and you and basically everybody else naturally run away from difficult and tedious things. Then, after we've run away, we're really good at justifying to ourselves that it was the right thing to do, never realizing how much harm we've potentially caused ourselves.*

Somebody you meet who doesn't buy from you didn't say no because they didn't like you. You didn't give them enough of a reason to buy. Consumers are consumers because they have pains they want to go away, itches they want scratched. If you make it easy for them to make a decision they feel is right for them — so the pain goes away — they'll be thankful. Stop complicating things. It doesn't help anybody.

Here's your unfair advantage: Learn how to differentiate yourself by highlighting a single aspect about you that stands out. This is not about gaining thousands of followers online. It's about appealing to a very small, very faithful community that believes in you (online or in-person). It's about establishing what we call at the Online Trainer Academy your 1% Uniqueness

---

* *There's a lot of talk in the behavioral economics field of study over whether humans are rational or irrational. We're neither.*

Humans are a post-rationalizing species. Most of what happens is driven by emotion or, as Nobel Prize-winning psychologist Daniel Kahneman calls it, System 1. The process (simplified) says that our unconscious and emotional brains drive action. But then System 2 (our clear-thinking, more rational brain) can't handle how little control it had over the process. It then proceeds to carve out a convenient post-rationalization justifying whatever happened by working backward and creating a nice-sounding narrative.

There's been lots written about this. If you want to know more, I strongly suggest going to the source with Kahneman's book, Thinking, Fast and Slow.

Factor.*

So ... this sounds good in theory, but what does it look like in action? Keep reading.

WHAT IS OTA?

*You'll hear me mention the Online Trainer Academy (OTA) a few times throughout this book. OTA is like getting a degree in online fitness business. Boasting the seminal textbook on the subject and with alumni in 83-plus countries, it's our flagship certification and mentorship program. Learn more at **theptdc.com/ota.***

Marketing medicine

Buckley's is a popular Canadian medicine with the tagline, "It tastes awful. And it works."

Red Bull is an energy drink that tastes like medicine. Its many competitors taste better, come in larger cans, cost less, and have the same stimulating ingredients (taurine, caffeine, vitamin B, sugar).

---

* *I'll talk about this more as this section continues, but by now you may be wondering how to pull this off. It all comes down to, in super-fancy technical terms, the idiosyncratic fit heuristic.*

Translation: The heuristic (rule of thumb) basically means, "If this is you, then this is for you."

The better you call out your ideal prospect and market your service specific to him, the easier his decision will be, and the easier a time you'll have making sales.

If you were to design a drink to compete with Coca Cola, the obvious path would be finding something that tastes better, comes in larger cans, and costs less. Red Bull is the opposite. It tastes horrible,* comes in a small can, and is outrageously expensive. Yet somehow, the company's sold 62 billion overpriced, undersized cans in 171 countries.

So what the heck is going on here? And how does this relate to fitness?

From what I understand, it'd be easy to make Buckley's and Red Bull taste good. The awful tastes are purposeful product decisions with marketing implications. For some reason, people believe anything medicinal needs to taste bad to work.** A borderline pain threshold is required as a type of placebo.

I refer to the pain threshold as a "demented theater," and it's proven necessary to sell not just medicine and amped-up vodka mixers but, well, just about everything.

---

*If you're one of the weirdos who thinks Red Bull tastes good, then know this: I think you're a weirdo.

** At time of writing, Buckley's is running a brilliant campaign in the Toronto subway system (the TTC) to celebrate the company's 100th anniversary.

Entire subway cars up and down are plastered with their ads. There are 100 panels in total. Each panel represents a different year and includes a person dressed from that era (1972, 1947, etc.), the bottle, an empty spoon, and the model making the face of someone who just drank something vile.

It's brilliant.

Case in point: exercise.

Exercise is simple. Jump up and down 50 times. That's your workout. The best fat loss exercise? Do something you suck at. The body burns more energy when it moves inefficiently. So run for fat loss if you suck at running, but know that once you become a moderately skilled runner, its fat-burning power decreases.

Nutrition is also simple. Eat tons of veggies, protein, a fair amount of fats, and high-quality carbs surrounding your workouts. Control intake of junk food and refined sugars.

The above are oversimplifications and don't take into account any special circumstances like disease, but I think most will agree that if the general population followed this oversimplified advice, society would be a lot healthier than it is.* And yet, few do it.

The problem with undifferentiated and simplified fitness and nutrition advice? No demented theater.

People need a reason to make a decision, to believe that one thing is better than something else.

Exercise is simple, but for people to begin and adhere to fitness programming, that programming needs to sound in some way special, complex, advanced, and, most of all, right for them. This is why the same physiological

---

For the majority of the sedentary and mostly sedentary population, it's really quite simple. Step one: Get them to move. How they move doesn't quite matter. Once they're moving, then you can start stressing the specifics.

principles of EPOC (Orange Theory) and low-carb dieting (keto) return to the spotlight marketed as a new breakthrough every five to 10 years with a slight twist. They can be made to sound fancy and advanced, and therefore, they sell.

The truth about "great" trainers

> *A great trainer doesn't have to design a great workout. She has to design a good enough workout and get her clients to want to do the workout.*

Marketing doesn't stop once a client pays you. In order to get a client amped about her program and engaged in the process, you've got to market the specific workout. Marketing never stops. Sorry to break it to all you do-gooder trainers who "just want to help people," but **the best trainers are better marketers than they are trainers.**

Before you get all worried that you suddenly have to have a master's degree in online marketing to make this business work, relax. In chapter three of the Online Trainer Academy's textbook, *The Fundamentals of Online Training*, I share the truth of online marketing:

> *"Another possible distraction waving its alluring bells and whistles at you is online marketing. While online marketing can be an asset — and we will cover the essentials in this program — the truth is, most trainers never have to use it.*

"I don't know everything about online marketing, but I know enough to know you can't really know everything about it. It's endlessly complex. That makes it perfectly suited for procrastinators because there's always one more thing you can do. It's a great recipe for getting stuck and never doing anything.

"Common online marketing strategies (email autoresponse systems, paid advertisements, setting up social media accounts, and more) may seem like the obvious choice for generating online clients. But through developing, testing, and refining this program, I discovered that there is a better way. In fact, of the thousands of people who have used this program, most have never needed to use online marketing."

In the Online Trainer Academy we mentor our students through the process of building a bulletproof online fitness business. Here, in this book, I can't mentor you directly (though I'd love to have you join us in OTA), but I can tell you what you need to know and what you can confidently ignore, both online and offline.

The same demented theater that requires Buckley's and Red Bull to taste awful — and fitness to be sold as more complicated than it is — is what makes *you* believe marketing needs to be complex. You don't need funnels, or secret scripts, or even paid advertising. You just need the basic skills.

In exercise, the basic skills are body awareness and motivation. If they're checked off, a client will achieve on any program as long as the workouts are "good enough" and performed with a reasonable level of intensity and consistency. For clients who aren't competing or don't have special needs, it all works.

In marketing, there are three basic and fundamental skills:

1. Productivity
2. Focus
3. A deep understanding of the core marketing principles

We'll talk in greater detail about these core principles in later chapters, but let's dig into a couple of basic truths first.

Strive for innovation, not improvement

The Japanese have a term called *kaizen*, which roughly translates to "continual improvement." About a gazillion fitness companies around the world have adopted the name. Sure, why not, sounds cool. After all, we're trained to improve, make things a little bit better day after day. But here's a secret: *Kaizen* is a fine model for achieving fitness goals, but a terrible model for building your business.

> *In marketing, you don't want improvement. You want innovation. You want quantum leaps, not baby steps.*

Bulletproof, the makers of Bulletproof Coffee, $10
chocolate bars, and a whole bunch of pricey foods and
products, innovated in the fitness industry just a few
years ago. The company has never disclosed its revenue
figures but has raised over $28 million in funding and
experienced incredible growth.

While the company has been controversial in fitness
circles due to their products' nutrition claims, you can't
help but admire their marketing acumen. As with any
case study, it's important to view the company and its
success as an objective outsider in order to learn. So
let's not be emotional about this. What can we learn
from Bulletproof?

Well, first of all, the company recognized the
marketability in information others saw and didn't
think was a big deal. Consider this:

- At the time of this writing, the Bulletproof®
  Upgraded™Coffee beans go for $14.99 per 12-ounce
  bag on their website.

- On Amazon, a 12-ounce bag of organic, fair trade
  coffee beans from a different brand retails for
  $7.45.

Bulletproof can charge two times more for their coffee
because the company claims that its upgraded coffee
has gone through a process to remove "mycotoxins."
Mycotoxins, put simply, are fungi. Two specific
types exist in coffee: Ochratoxin A and Aflatoxin B1.
Mycotoxins likely cause inflammation, fatigue, and

possibly cancer. Ample research backs up the claim. The stuff is nasty. It's also true that these fungi are present in most coffee. These upgraded beans seem like an obvious choice.

The catch? Coffee growers have known about mycotoxins for years and have been actively controlling and removing them. Not only that, but government health organizations have been closely monitoring the levels of these fungi in coffee beans imported into Canada, the United States, and many other countries around the world for decades.

In their book *Coffee: Physiology*, published in 1988 (decades before Bulletproof Coffee existed), authors R.J. Clarke and R. Macrae said it best: "Mycotoxins have sometimes been associated with coffee: here again their importance should not be dramatized as they do not present an undue toxicological hazard with the good manufacturing practices normally encountered in coffee production."

In short, mycotoxins are not an issue at all. You'll only find them in nonhazardous microdoses in any commercially available coffee in developed countries. Coffee growers were aware of the problem and adjusted their agricultural and manufacturing processes to fix it; they just didn't recognize the *marketability* of it. Bulletproof did, and used it to sell their coffee at two times the market price.

From the Sufi monasteries of Yemen in the 15th

century to today, coffee consumption has been a thing.
Some 500-plus years into the product cycle, Bulletproof
was still able to profit mightily from innovative
marketing based on information available to anybody.
The company made their own market. So, if you think
everything's already been done in the fitness industry,
let this be a lesson.

Find friendly waters

By now you may have heard of *Blue Ocean Strategy*,
by W. Chan Kim and Renée Mauborgne. In the book,
the authors describe the marketing landscape as two
oceans, one red and the other blue.

The red ocean is overcrowded, where most people are,
and where constant fighting for the same customers
leaves the water bloody and full of scavengers. There
are so many people doing the same things to attract
the same people that no one stands out. Competition
is rampant and eventually everybody competes and
underprices each other out of business.

The blue ocean is different. It's calm, open, and
uncharted. When you find (or better yet, create) a blue
ocean, you own it. It allows you to be a category of one.
In your blue ocean, when a lead comes in, you're the
market leader and control the conversation. No one
fights you for the lead because no one can.

Marc-André Seers, an online coach in Châteauguay,
Quebec, knows the benefit of being in a blue ocean. As

a bilingual coach, he could've marketed his services in either French or English. Most would have said English was the smarter choice. The market is bigger and English speakers are more accustomed to buying fitness services online. Most bilingual coaches like himself did the (not-so) smart thing and promoted themselves in English.

Marc-André saw a blue ocean: The decision to offer his services in French seemed scary at the time, but not only is he now making more money than he ever dreamed of, with 90 online clients, but he's taken his business completely online so he can travel the world.*

Successful trainers understand that true innovation means developing what makes them special. Instead of trying to offer slightly better service to the same clients as everybody else (and becoming increasingly frustrated that nobody cares), they know they need to present themselves differently. They find their angles, like Bulletproof did, and market those angles even if they aren't the first to come across the information.

Another thing: Once you find your blue ocean, don't move around. Stay there. Float. It takes time to foster community, build a reputation, and establish a premium position in that market. Think about how you can create something that's already popular and innovate it in a way that resonates. How? Play around with the concept of an intangible element — something

---

* Learn more about Marc here: **theptdc.com/marc.**

in your product or marketing that stands out, gets talked about, and puts you in a category of one.

For Starbucks, it's the language used to order. For Bulletproof, it's the stick of butter in the coffee (like it or not, it gets people talking). For my operation, the Online Trainer Academy, the intangible element is the textbook. Sure, the textbook is a tangible object thick enough to hurt someone if you whapped them on the head. But what the textbook contains, and represents, and ultimately delivers is our secret sauce to differentiation when marketing OTA.

Lots of people have created online courses to teach fit pros business practices, and a few others produced courses about online training. The program we created is unquestionably the best training program and mentorship in the world. I know it to be true and so do our alumni. But do you believe me? Maybe. Probably not. Anybody can say that they are the best and many do.

The Fundamentals of Online Training textbook is the intangible element communicating unconsciously that there was a tremendous amount of thoughtfulness and dedication put into curriculum development. Textbooks are extremely time-consuming and expensive to produce and print and ship. As a result, having one as part of the program says more than words ever could.

This innovation established the Online Trainer

Academy as a category of one, and I created a blue ocean for myself. Immediately it showed, without me having to say a thing, that the OTA certification and business development course was more thorough, more thoughtful, and more complete than anything else available.

I'll never forget what Charles "Petey" Bell, the owner of First Klass Nutrition in Bryant, Arkansas, said to me during an interview when asked why he decided to enroll in the OTA: "I hadn't really heard of you but I came across the materials and saw the book and thought to myself, *Ain't nobody going to go to so much trouble for some bulls*** course.*"

He's right.

How do you know when you've innovated successfully? When your customers tell you they never considered hiring or buying from anybody else.

Do you know what your clients really want?

"Professor Dumbledore. Can I ask you something?"

"Obviously, you've just done so," Dumbledore smiled. *"You may ask me one more thing, however."*

"What do you see when you look in the mirror?"

> *"I? I see myself holding a pair of thick, woolen socks." Harry stared.*
>
> *"One can never have enough socks," said Dumbledore. "Another Christmas has come and gone and I didn't get a single pair. People will insist on giving me books."*

In the Harry Potter saga, the Mirror of Erised shows a person's "deepest, most desperate desire." Dumbledore was probably lying to Harry about what he saw to protect a painful truth. Still, he made clear the point that he didn't want people to give him books.

For the head of the school, books seem like they're an obvious gift. But Dumbledore doesn't want books. He wants socks.

If you've ever claimed "the people I know aren't willing to invest in their fitness," then I have a hard truth for you: **People around you *are* willing to invest in their fitness. They just aren't willing to invest in *you*.** Why? You're giving them books when they want socks. You aren't selling them what they truly want.

Go beyond the surface level. Look deeper into the desires, and the fears, of your customer to know the true value of what you're selling. It's not really fat loss, or muscle gain (where's the innovation there?). It's definitely not health. It starts with *transformation* — the prospect is not happy with some part of themselves and thinks that there's happiness on the other side of that transformation. But it goes even deeper than that.

What is your prospect's past experience with transformation? **In almost every case, she will have tried and failed to accomplish the very thing that you're promising to help her achieve.** As a result, they lack belief not in the information or the process, but in themselves. Give her that belief in herself — and, in turn, you — and she'll buy.

A prospect needs to believe that you're the expert and that you have the solution for them.

Selling belief is your job. Without it, you'll never have an opportunity to coach fitness and nutrition.

Revisiting the 31-word marketing lesson

To start this book I shared 31 words that cover everything you need to know about marketing. Here it is again:

> *People don't want cheap, they want easy. They want perceived innovation, not slight improvement. And people don't want the best, they want to trust that whatever they are buying isn't crap.*

To bring this introduction to a close, let's deconstruct this short, yet powerful, passage line by line.

"People don't want cheap, they want easy."

The idea seems to fly in the face of logic. Ask people what they want and they say, "Low prices!" That's just common sense.

The best product at the best price always gets the sale, right? Nope, sorry, wrong.

Why, in this case (and so many others), is the customer wrong?

Because of false positives.

False positives come up in any survey of customers or prospects. When you ask questions in a public forum, you hear from two categories of people:

1. The boisterous few, whose opinions drown out the desires of the quiet many.
2. Those expressing false desires for the sake of appearances.

To the second point, consider the natural herding behavior of humans. We all crave perceived social standing in a community. As a result, our actions inside a community don't necessarily represent what we truly want. Instead, they are representations of *how we want to appear*. We say that we want things because we feel like it's what a high-status member of the tribe *should* want.

In other words, people say they want something because they think it makes them look good to want it. And often, they don't want it (or don't want it bad enough to pay for it).

This explains why some trainers create products or programs that people say they want, but nobody buys. It's not because they hate or don't respect the trainer, and it's certainly not because the prospect isn't willing to "invest in fitness." It happens, simply, because the trainer was led astray by false positives.

I know your reaction to that might be, "Wait, hold on. How am I supposed to know when I'm *not* supposed to listen to what prospects tell me?"

Fair question. The answer: Asking "what do you want from training" is designed to elicit a surface answer that probably sounds logical but isn't deep-down true for that person.

Why? Almost every prospect who comes to you with a fitness goal has tried to achieve it before. They've either failed, or succeeded a bit before they relapsed. You're not selling these clients a program. You're selling the confidence that they can achieve the transformation they've been failing to achieve.

The majority of fitness consumers couldn't care less if a program is the best or the cheapest. Prospects only care that they have a problem (they don't like the way they look, they have poor health, etc.) and want the problem to go away as quickly and as easily as possible. They don't want cheap, they want easy.

The easier we make it for a client to find us, contact us,
get just enough of the info they need, and start working
with us, the better the chance that the client will buy.

"They want perceived innovation, not slight improvement."

We've already talked about this. Present your services
as innovation, not improvement.

You must establish your own category, making you the
obvious choice and rendering price irrelevant.[*]

"And people don't want the best, they want to trust that whatever they're buying isn't crap."

There's a concept in behavioral psychology called *loss
aversion*, defined simply as "losses loom larger than
gains." This means people have a tendency to put much
more energy into avoiding a loss than acquiring a gain.

The majority of purchase decisions are the result
of something called *satisficing* — a decision-making
heuristic that entails searching through the available
alternatives until an acceptability threshold is met.

The reason that we buy (and pay more for) brands is
not that we believe they're better. We buy because we're

---

[*] *Never make up new physiological or biomechanical principles; that
would be dishonest. Instead, innovate by branding a principle uniquely.
Present a prospect with an opportunity that resonates with them in a new
way. A new name, hook, or angle is often enough.*

more sure they aren't crap. Unconsciously, we're aware brands have invested a lot into their product and, as a result, they have more to lose by selling a bad product. In a sense, a strong brand provides consumers with a shortcut to reach their acceptability purchase threshold and, because they've made our decision easier, we pay more and buy more readily from them.

Bringing it home: Why buy fitness when you can get it for free?

After all this, there's a simple answer to this question. I wrote about it in my first book, *Ignite the Fire*, back in 2011 and it's more true today than ever.

The answer is that fitness doesn't have value unless you create it. But when you do create it, you can change lives. As a result, as I've said time and time again,

People buy trainers, not training.

In other words, it comes down to you. Yes, you. People are buying you. Not the workout. Not the nutrition plan. Not the product, pill, or potion. They're buying you. They're buying your brand. They're buying the reason why you do what you do.

This introduction scratched the surface on key concepts, primarily you establishing yourself and your brand as an obvious choice for prospects, and the rest of the book will give you dozens of ways you can do that, beginning with the eight blind spots holding you back from getting the clients you deserve. Let's go there now.

PART ONE

How to Get More People to Buy from You

CHAPTER 1

8 Blind Spots Holding You Back from Getting the Clients You Deserve

"Many of life's failures are people who did not

realize how close they were to success when

they gave up."

—*Thomas Edison*

If you've ever said "I didn't even know I was doing it wrong," then you're in the majority. Blind spots. Everybody's got 'em.

Let's talk about some of the biggest blind spots when it comes to getting clients. Two pieces of advice before we begin:

1. **Open your mind.** A closed mind in itself is a blind

spot. Be ready for new ideas.

2. **Be patient.** Give yourself time to process and implement in smart ways, not just as-soon-as-friggin'-possible-preferably-yesterday.

As you read about the eight blind spots, you'll see what I mean.

Blind spot #1: You have a limited definition of "communication"

Whatever historians (or hipsters) will call this era 100 years from now — the information age, the internet age, the insanity age — you just know that every think piece written about it will kick off with some form of "the entire planet became interconnected within a few short years, making a small world even smaller."

It's true. Communication is easier than ever. Thirty years ago, a phone in everyone's pocket still seemed very *Star Trek*. That smartphone keeping your butt cheek warm features more than a dozen ways to communicate with loved ones, colleagues, clients, and total strangers: text, FaceTime and other video call apps, email, social (lots of platforms), mobile web content, and oh yeah, phone (how quaint).

Unfortunately, a lot of people think "communication" begins and ends with their smartphone. And their definition of "communication" is limited because they've allowed their imaginations to be limited.

Let's bust out of that rut. Ask yourself:

- Am I communicating with as many people as I can daily?
- How am I communicating?
- What am I communicating?
- Do I have a plan? Do I know *why* I do all the things I do in this area?

For years I've gotten a variation of the same question at least once a day. It always looks something like this:

> *"I've tried everything. I have my website set up and I'm sending out Facebook ads and can't get any clients. How are you guys getting clients?"*

Before trying to dissect what the problem is with their advertising, or website, or funnel, I always ask the same thing: **"How many people have you spoken to today?"**

Crickets. Or maybe someone says, "Um, I dunno." Or "Nobody, I guess." Or my favorite, "What do you mean by 'spoken to'?"

The truth? Paid advertising and funnels and headlines and that stuff are gasoline on the fire. They're powerful. But they aren't where you start.

Trying to figure out the best Facebook ad that works *right now* is no way to get clients. Even if you're able to figure out how to "master" Facebook advertising today, things will change tomorrow and you're going to be forced to reinvent yourself. That's one pointless hamster wheel, trust me.

Paid ads are a tactic, nothing less and nothing more. I'm not against them. I use them. They simply don't come first. What does? *Talking to people.* As in, verbally, with your lips, tongue, and voice. Face to face whenever possible. Yes, in our beloved information age driven by our warm and precious smartphones, talking to people is the best way to build unbelievable relationships and trust.

Here's the easiest way to do it: Have a conversation with at least five new people every day.

Anabela Souto, the owner of Nutriessence Fitness, tried it as an experiment and it quickly became not just a habit, but a business driver. "I love this. I now have seven new personal training clients just from talking to people. It works."

The easiest way to get into it is make the process a ritual. Put five paper clips on the right side of your computer. After you have a conversation, move one to the left side of the computer. Once all paper clips have shifted, you're done for the day. Repeat the next.

THE PROBLEM WITH PAID ADS ON SOCIAL MEDIA

Social media ad platforms have gotten easier to use and, surprise, more people use them. This means not only will ads get more expensive over time, but users are going to get more and more accustomed to seeing them. And ignoring them.

Not good, and definitely not something to stake your success on. Don't believe me? When was the last time you bought anything purely from an advertisement on social media? What do you think when you see an ad from somebody about something you've never heard of?

That's right, you don't think. You ignore. That's the point. Very few people purchase anything from any company after seeing a random advertisement fly through their feed anymore. Advertising combined with other brand and product development pieces all working together ... now we're talking!

Paid advertising on social media can be a huge boon to your business, but only if you're dialed in on your message, market, and audience in addition to knowing your numbers (how much you can pay to acquire a lead based on how much a lead is worth to you).

Because it's gotten so much more competitive, paid advertising by itself is no longer a feasible way to run a business. It must be combined with a strong back end of profitable, high-margin *products and/or services to sell.*

Social media has changed the world of marketing, but while everything has changed, nothing is different. Relationships, reputation, lifetime customer value (LCV), and referrals are where it's at.

So paid ads on social media aren't bad, but they're not the end-all. Instead, they must be part of a bigger strategy. Lucky for you, we'll talk all about that later in this book.

That's just one way to change your approach to "communication." See what I mean about opening your mind? Later in the book, we'll go deeper into the other problems in this blind spot, like knowing how and why you communicate certain things to prospects, how you present yourself to the world, and the value of positive interaction. After all, good communication leads to great reputation. And that's invaluable in this business.

Blind spot #2: You have the wrong marketing mindset

Twentieth-century department store magnate John Wanamaker had a great take on advertising: "Half the money I spend on advertising is wasted. The trouble is I don't know which half." Truer words, you know? Too many trainers think marketing means spending money.

You spend a little cash on ads or some other expensive marketing trick, and despite a few metrics and maybe some feedback, you have no idea if those dollars are working.

Let's get technical for a moment. Advertising spend can be measured a few ways, but the most common is a metric called "cost per impression (CPI)" or, on the internet, cost per 1,000 impressions (CPM).*

This doesn't mean that 1,000 people pay attention to your message, just that it appeared on their screen at some point. The goal is to get your CPM as low as possible while maintaining lead quality.

Now, you could do this a few ways. The most common highlights the biggest mistake a lot of marketers make: single, narrow-minded thinking.

An example of bad thinking: If I want to get my CPM down, I need to send a bit better ad with a bit better headline, or picture, or targeting, or description. This is fine, and it might help you out in the short-term, but you're still going to lose.

Here's a better mindset: To maximize CPM, take a two-pronged approach where you build a brand people want to hear from and you craft a business model where you pay once and get impressions for years. Sounds

---

CPM is the most common, but there are a host of other ways to measure the effectiveness of advertising. Cost Per Conversion and Cost Per Click (both referred to as CPC) are both used as well. And this is just for direct response advertising. Brand advertising is a totally different beast. For now, for us, CPM is good enough.

great, right? It's cost effective and low maintenance after the initial effort. So what kinds of things get these kinds of results?

Reputation does. So does great content (you create it once and it's costly to produce but can result in thousands of impressions on an ongoing basis). While I'm obviously bullish on content, it's not 100 percent necessary. There is one other way ...

For eight years, I spent very little on conventional paid advertising while still generating millions of dollars in profits. Instead of paying for clicks, most of my marketing budget went to sending gifts and building relationships. I view this as a way to get a disproportionately positive response for the time and money invested.

Think about it: If I can send somebody a beautiful gift that costs me $20 that they see multiple times a day, every day, for a year, how many impressions will that gift provide versus that same $20 spent on a paid ad?

Want a totally random yet illustrative example? Give a welcome mat to a customer. That customer steps on it every time she enters or exits her house. So do guests who comment on the welcome mat. Guess what happens next? The person who bought the welcome mat (you) comes up in conversation.

I'm not just talking about this stuff. It's what I do.

OTA grad Carolina Belmares is crushing it right now. In

addition to meshing the Precision Nutrition ProCoach Software with the business development tools in the Online Trainer Academy, Carolina has a full stable of online clientele and recently took her whole family on a vacation to Mexico. Super cool. She's also building a reputation as an expert with her own network of coaches who respect her.

Carolina loves tacos. So I got her a welcome mat that says in big letters, YOU BETTER HAVE TACOS. The mat found a home at the front entrance of Carolina's house for more than a year. Every time she left or entered, she thought of me. Every time she had a guest over (a colleague, friend, etc.) the mat, and I, came up in conversations.

How much business did that one gift directly generate for me? I have no idea. Maybe nothing. Or maybe a lot. In the ensuing years, Carolina became one of our biggest promotional partners for the Online Trainer Academy so it couldn't have hurt. But if you follow my logic up until now, then you can surely see the theory I'm laying out backs up the maxim:

Not everything that can be counted counts.

Not everything that counts can be counted. *

Now, maybe you're thinking, *that's cute,* or *okay, yeah,*

---

* *This is commonly attributed to Albert Einstein but it probably shouldn't be. (If you trust the internet, basically every quote originated with either Abraham Lincoln or Albert Einstein.) The most appropriate attribution for this quote is to the sociologist William Bruce Cameron.*

fun, but I want you to think differently. Ask, "How many dollars would I have to spend on an advertisement to get that number of impressions?" *This* is how your thinking should go.

Ignore the incessant noise, and ignore the ads that try to get you to pay to learn the "latest" best secret for getting clients. Play the long game, think differently, act differently. Enrich your reputation and you enrich yourself.

Trust and reputation are an impression game. The more times that people come across your name in a positive light, the more they trust you.* Attempting to purchase those impressions is costly. This is a better way.

Yes, engaging with people takes work. If it were easy to get platoons of clients just by firing off an ad, everybody would do it. I've been doing this since 2011, an eternity in internet years. In that time, I've seen countless fitness pros come and go and almost as many fitness business coaches disappear.

Why did they all fail, give up, and leave? They never

---

* *Jacoby and Kelley's study published in 1989 in the* Journal of Personality and Social Psychology *titled "Becoming Famous Overnight: Limits on the Ability to Avoid Unconscious Influences of the Past" is useful to better understand the all-important "sleeper effect" that describes the power of multiple impressions over time on establishing authority, credibility, trust, and reputation.*

Spoiler alert: They literally made up names of people who don't exist and, through a series of manipulated exposures, research participants not only said these fake people existed, but that they'd heard of them and they were famous.

took the time to build relationships with readers and customers and didn't understand the fundamentals of CPI and how it relates.

Blind spot #3: You don't study the past

I recently read an old marketing book in which the author argued that "the internet" presents a lot of moneymaking opportunities — particularly with something that industry pundits referred to as "on-line marketing."

Yeah, that internet has some potential, right? Pardon me while I go on-line.

We live in an age where everything is new, yet nothing is different. I read a lot and can say most books written about marketing in the last 10 years aren't worth the time it would take to open them. They're full of rehashed ideas, hacked together haphazardly, with a bunch of stories thrown in for good measure.

Truth: It's too easy to do a bad job with marketing these days, and that's why most people suck at it. In fact, most trainers are lazy, ignorant, negligent marketers, which is why you can blast past them with the littlest know-how and effort.

For this reason, I've made a habit of seeking out marketing tomes written before the internet existed. They're fascinating and useful.

Before the internet, marketing was harder. Missing the

mark had real consequences. Sending a failed mailing could cost tens of thousands of dollars. Both the cost of entry and price of failure were higher and, as a result, marketers were forced to be good.

I put my books and many of my promotional pieces into print. Why? The finality and hard cost force quality. With print, I can't tweak a status update, resend an email because I missed including a link, or make an edit to an ebook because I screwed up an important point.

I'm not necessarily suggesting you put your work into print. It depends on your situation. What I am suggesting is that you approach your marketing with that print mindset, as if you're paying to send it and can't change it when you do.

Imagine how much more effort you would put into composing your emails and choosing your mail list if you had to pay for a stamp for every message sent to every person like you would a letter.

Imagine how much more time you would invest into considering every touchpoint, every additional revenue opportunity, every upsell, and every add-on if you had to pay *every single time* you communicated with your potential customers.

Imagine how much better you would be forced to be.

That's the mindset I want you to bring to your marketing.

And to show you that this isn't some abstract concept,

I'll tell you the story of how I and my team used this mindset to launch our *Fitness Marketing Monthly* collection in 2018.

WHAT'S FMM?

We published 10 issues and more than 200,000 words of next-level marketing content for fitness pros in FMM. Now you can get every single word in one beautiful package, Fitness Marketing Monthly: The Complete Collection. *The potent collection was so impressive that* Entrepreneur *magazine dedicated a full-page feature to its production and completion in their June 2019 issue. Check out* **theptdc.com/fmm** *if you want a master class in fitness marketing.*

When it came time to launch FMM, we had to craft a promotion program to get the word out. We needed to make a splash without spending a fortune.

Here's what we did:

- Sent 5,000 VERY SPECIAL targeted direct mail packages.
- Wrote a sales page that had marketing experts across all industries salivating.
- Fired up our two Facebook groups about the promotion.
- Carefully crafted an email sequence.

What's more interesting, and more educational, is what we *didn't* do:

- Create a single piece of audio or video. So I guess you don't *have* to do video after all, eh?
- Overspend. We spent only $5,000 on paid digital advertising. This was almost entirely retargeting. We did not use paid ads for lead generation.
- Show the actual product.

Think about that last point for a second: *Not a single person had seen the actual product.*

The lesson: The importance of what you're selling pales in comparison to your ability to highlight the problem it solves and paint the picture of the transformation you are providing to your customer.

Your clients don't care what's in your program. The details are irrelevant. How many sessions, how much support, how often you send the program, the sets, the reps, and all of that ... none of it matters if you craft your sales and value propositions properly and get results that, over time, speak for themselves.

Before the first issue was shipped, 1,615 subscribers opted in at $39.97 per month, many of them paying for a full year up front. That's $774,618.60 in added revenue. By the time the project completed, FMM generated $1.2 million in revenue with $456,000 profit (rounded-off numbers). Our cost to market was tiny because we approached it with a level of seriousness you rarely see in this day and age. Because of this, we were able to invest a lot more money into the production, creating a beautiful, world-class product.

Everything is different and nothing is new

I took down a few notes while reading that comically outdated marketing book that prove *nothing is new*. The principles are the principles. All three of the bullets below are currently being marketed as *NEW* and *IMPORTANT* because of all the changes happening with *scary algorithms*:

1. The author speaks about how expensive it is to acquire a customer in the 1990s and, as a result, a strong back-end system of selling products and additional profits centers needs to be added onto the original purchase. *My note: Acquiring customers is expensive. Once acquired, spend your money keeping and selling to existing customers.*
2. You cannot win by marketing in only one channel. A customer needs to hear about you in multiple places. *My note: Focus on one channel so as not to dilute your efforts and then distribute that person to other communication methods or media.*
3. Every business should include a source of revenue from selling information. It's the easiest and cheapest way to acquire customers at break-even (or profit) and pad the bottom line. *My note: Every trainer should have an information marketing business.*

People are people and respond to the same types of

marketing, value propositions, and sales techniques that they always have. Nothing has changed. But maybe one thing should: Nowadays communication is free and immediate and this has made us terrible communicators.

Here's a thought experiment: What if you took $1 of your hard-earned cash and put it into a jar for every individual email that you sent? Would self-imposing a fixed cost on every email you send make you a better, more thoughtful, more complete communicator?

I wonder.

Blind spot #4: You ask lousy questions

You want to get better at your business. But you have questions. Maybe you think about hiring a fitness business coach or some kind of consultant.

Know what? You don't need to hire anyone. At least not yet. Information is abundant and (mostly) free. You can learn anything you want but it requires one fundamental skill: *You must be able to ask good questions.* Bad questions yield answers that can have detrimental consequences. The worst information, after all, is bad information. And, oh my, these days, my friend, there's a lot of bad information out there! Once you understand the question you need to ask, then you can seek out a mentor or coach.

My company runs multiple communities with tens

of thousands of coaches in each. They are true communities with abundance mindsets where everybody wants each other to succeed. If you want help with a specific issue you're having with a client, or marketing, or anything else, you can get it in there.

But we can only help if you ask a good question. "I'm looking to get started with online training. Any tips?" won't get you anywhere. It's a waste of your time to write it, and a waste of anybody else's time to answer. Most won't.

Tell me *why* you want to start online training, what you've been doing previously, and who you want to train. The more specific you are with your question, the better the answer because there is no one best way.

Pretend you've only got one shot at this. Pretend you're going to put a stamp on your Facebook post, send it off in the mail, and have to wait six weeks to (hopefully) get a response.

If you pretend this process is harder, you'll be better.

Blind spot #5: You don't know who your ideal client is

When you're just starting out, you might think, *I'll take all comers*, and sign up anyone. You want income, growth, and the feeling that you're doing well in the business. And that approach might work in the very beginning, but let me tell you, the key to long-term success is identifying who you *truly* want to train.

Why? Think of it this way: If you can't stand kids, you shouldn't be training youth sports groups. If you can't connect with older people, you shouldn't be training senior citizens. Mismatched clients and trainers drive each other insane. Even if you try to force it, you'll end up unhappy and that leads to bad results for you *and* your client.

But an ideal client? Imagine someone paying you who ...

- Shares your interests.

- Values your expertise.

- Knows that you can solve her problems.

- Becomes a raving fan who refers others to you.

Once you identify your ideal client, you can then adjust your marketing efforts to appeal directly to those folks, which makes client acquisition that much easier. Eventually you'll become known as The One to that group of people, and you'll be the obvious choice when those folks look for a trainer.

How do you identify your ideal client? Easy. Use this worksheet to create your fictional "ideal" and watch how this person instantly takes shape ...

Client name: _____

Age/Gender: _____

Job/Income: _____

Training history: _____

Favorite sport: _____

Stated fitness goal: _____

Secret, real fitness goal: _____

Biggest struggle: _____

What gets him/her out of bed each morning:_____

Other interests: _____

The more you know about your clients, the better you can target everything from marketing to coaching cues to celebrating goals. The more you understand their fears, frustrations, desires, goals — and how you'll help solve them — the better results you'll get. And think about this: If you have mutual interests and really connect, your client won't be missing workouts and will be more enthusiastic about your program.

Push for empathy. Try to think and feel as they do. What interests them outside the gym? What's bothering them? What are they dealing with? You don't have to be anyone's BFF, but connecting on a level above trainer/ client will benefit you both.

Blind spot #6: You don't know how many clients you need

When you combine numbers with dreams, it's easy to screw up the math. For example, maybe you have a number in mind representing what you believe is the perfect amount of clients or revenue. It's the scenario you dreamed about when you decided to become a trainer. "If I just get to X, everything will be awesome."

The problem is X is a random number. You based it on something you heard, or someone else's business, or some other out-of-thin-air metric that sounded good. But if you say 50 clients is your perfect number, or 15, or 35, how do you know? What did you base your math on? Fifty is just as arbitrary a number as, say, 46 or 52. It's just round and looks impressive.

You need to figure out how many clients you *really* need. Define it, because when you do, you'll probably realize the number is a lot smaller than you thought.

If that's true, then it's also probably true that all you need is a good referral system to thrive. You need a product, traffic, and a conversion mechanism, of course. But once you nail that down, it's a matter of optimizing each one — not adding in other stuff. Knowing exactly how many clients you need saves you time, money, and effort. It sets your business down in real terms: *Here's what it needs to work.*

So let's talk some fourth-grade math. First, you need to calculate your freedom number.* I talk a lot about the freedom number because it's truly one of the foundations of a successful training business. Your freedom number is the amount of income you need to live comfortably each month (remember, we're not angling to "get by" or "muddle through").

Start by tallying up the amount of money per month, after taxes, that you need to fulfill your basic needs: rent, food, funds to care for others (if applicable), and a small amount for extravagance.

Now figure your "continued funds," the money you're making either passively or by doing what you love to do. In other words, it's money made through work you want to continue doing. (For example, suppose you're taking your business online but still want to train 10 ideal clients in the gym. You would calculate how much you make from those 10 clients each month and use that as the "continued funds" number.)

Your freedom number = Essentials - Continued funds

Your freedom number is the difference between what

---

* *You may have seen this from me before. If not, you'll surely see it again. This concept is so valuable that it's repeated in almost every one of my books and products. It forms the base of your business.*

you need to make to survive and how much you're making doing the work you want to continue doing. It gives you an earnings target each month.

Now, some more math. How much do you charge a client per month? See where I'm going? If you divide your freedom number by the amount you charge the average client, you arrive at the minimum number of clients you need to cover your freedom number.

That's just the minimum, mind you. You can adjust upward or downward depending on changes in what you charge, or how much bandwidth you have for more clients beyond the minimum.

So that's why I said your "dream" number of clients was a random mirage. You need to do this simple math to figure out how many clients you truly need to thrive as a trainer. It probably won't be a nice, round, impressive number. But it's a number you need to know.

Then, once you get there, you're free. And freedom is providing yourself the opportunity to fail. By knowing the number, you know when you can comfortably take risks and you'll also know how much money you have to reinvest back into personal development and your business. This is when the fun really starts.

Blind spot #7: You're not following up enough

It was overcast outside the gym where I worked. A

client canceled last minute, which presented me with an hour to kill. Par for the course. Still, I was bored. Good thing I always had a book in my gym bag. *A day like any other*, I thought.

Then the garbage man showed up.

"This a gym?" he asked. Big guy. Italian. Barrel chest. His voice was booming, confident, and authoritative.

"Yup," I replied.

We spoke for a while and he told me he owned a trash management company. Said he needed to lose some weight.

I felt like I had a lucky charm up my butt. He wanted to start three times per week, could train anytime, and was going to buy 50 sessions.

"Just didn't bring my credit card," he said. "I'll call tomorrow."

He didn't call.

I followed up and left a message. A week passed. I called again and left a message. No response.

I put him on a list to call once a month, just to check in. Every month we phoned him. Most of the time we got the answering machine. Once he picked up and said that he was busy and would call back right away because he was interested. He didn't. On more than one occasion, he did call back and booked in an appointment to sign up.

He never showed.

What would you do after three months of this? I know most people would write him off. But let me tell you, impatience with prospects like him is a huge mistake.

There are three types of leads: fast, medium, and slow.

Many marketing systems focus on fast-lane clients because doing so gets immediate, seemingly overnight results. Whenever you hear a person say, "I just did this one thing and I got X number of clients," they're referring to fast-lane clients. Nothing wrong with it, but there is a limited number of these people and, for most, it's too small a number. So yes, skim the cream off the top. Just don't stop there.

The need for instant gratification runs deep, which means you've likely seen (and hopefully not been charmed by) bad business coaches promoting amazing results in almost no time. These people aren't teaching marketing. They're teaching glorified order-taking. It works for a very short period of time to convert the fast-lane clients and then completely falls flat.

Here's the reality:

- Three to five percent are fast-lane leads.
- Five to 10 percent are medium.
- 80 to 90 percent are slow.

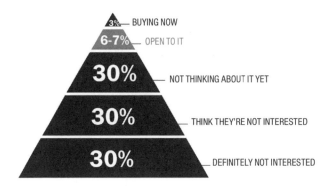

At any point in time, 80-90% of leads simply aren't interested. This doesn't mean that they won't ever be and it's important to stay top of mind so that you get the business when they decide it's time to buy. (Image adapted from The Fundamentals of Online Training *textbook that accompanies the* Online Trainer Academy Certification and Mentorship. *Learn more: **theptdc.com/ota.**)*

Ignore this and you miss out on 80 to 90 percent of leads. You may have some immediate "wins," but you'll lose long-term, wondering how Jimmy the Trainer over there has a business that seems to grow every month while yours sputters, spits, and suffers.

Go ahead and convert the fast lane. Take out the low-hanging fruit. All that you generally need to do is make an offer and get it in front of the right people.

Then the serious work starts. The work that requires pig-headed discipline. Systems for following up. Consistency. And if you're not willing to put in the work now, you have no chance.

Gavyn Berntsen, owner of Start Afresh Exercise and

Nutrition Coaching in Auckland, New Zealand, knows all about the hidden value in the slow lane. After following the module in the Online Trainer Academy about pig-headed discipline, complete with email scripts for reconnecting with old clients, he got to work.

According to Gavyn, "I've had nearly 100 old clients who I'd just lost touch with, and hadn't followed up with. I sent out 100-ish emails wishing them a happy new year and a line unique to each client. Almost immediately had four replies thanking me for following up, letting me know that they were ready to start training again soon and wanted new programs. In a nutshell, just follow up with lost contacts. They actually want to hear from you."

Meanwhile, eight months after that gloomy day, my garbage man showed up to say that he was ready, credit card in hand. He paid $4,463.50 up front and booked three sessions a week moving forward. Good thing I kept following up the entire time or else he would have gone elsewhere.

Blind spot #8: You forget to keep it simple

Canada's cold in the winter, so my family and I make a habit of escaping to someplace warm, which leads to some wonderful adventures ... and some unforgettable misadventures. In 2018, we lived in a town called Sosua in the Dominican Republic and in our final two weeks we had to:

- Evacuate our hotel in the Dominican Republic as it was getting destroyed by high ocean swells.
- Scramble to find a new hotel in the D.R.
- Return to Toronto after five months abroad.

All of this with a one-year-old toddler.

Those two weeks felt like I was being pulled in a thousand different directions. I recalled the old Chinese term for a type of torture: *Lingchi.* In English it can mean a number of things ... *the lingering death ... the slow slicing ... death by a thousand cuts.*

The truth is, even as my adopted home was being destroyed by the ocean and my family and I hurriedly packed our things, not knowing where we would sleep that night, my business kept on ticking.

Every week since, as I was getting on planes, or planning the following winter's itinerary, packing, traveling, setting up house in new lands, and generally living the life I want to live, my business kept on ticking.

My wife and I enjoyed four to six months abroad for seven years straight (two of them with a baby). We've lived in Costa Rica, the Dominican Republic, Thailand, Indonesia, Greece, Montenegro, Mexico, Hawaii, and Uruguay, and visited about 20 other countries in the process. All of this happened while I was growing and running an international publishing business.

When I have time to reflect on all the crazy times we've

had, all I can think about is how important it is to build a robust business, one that is immune to outside influence, one that can withstand even a thousand cuts.

So many trainers try to do too much, and end up getting nothing done. This modern obsession with omnipresence leads to an absorption in the small, silly things like thinking you need to be everywhere, answering every message, showing up at every event, and documenting your life to anybody who happens across your platform.

Creating content is invaluable. But it's gotta be *really good*. Content is abundant. Good content that's produced in a consumable way is scarce.

The bigger your ambitions are, the simpler your plan must be. The structure of my business is simple. It's taken many years to rip away the fluff. I speak negatively about complicated funnels, depending on paid advertising as your sole source for lead generation, and long, rambling email autoresponse sequences because I've done it all.

There are lots of stories I've never told, like the one where I wrote 100 emails for an autoresponse sequence we internally referred to as "the money tree." The intelligence built into the automation was brilliant. We built more than 40 income streams into it. It got published and it worked. For a while it was beautiful. I was living the dream, right?

The problem: It was too complicated. It would've

worked for a few more months, maybe even a year
or two, but, over time, I slowly lost control over the
system and pissed off too many subscribers. Tech
changed and so did the market. So the money tree was
scrapped. Months of work. A hundred emails. Some of
it got repurposed. Most of it went in the trash.

This is one example of overly complex things I did on
my journey to simplification. Because we don't need
more content, or more businesses haphazardly slapped
together. What we need are more eloquent business
structures painfully produced with purpose.

It's easy to think of complicated ways to do something.
Fun even. But once it's time for the doing, death by
a thousand cuts is common. Beginners complicate,
experts simplify. Simplification is way harder than
complication. It requires a lot more work.

And perhaps that's what we need.

PERHAPS WE NEED A BIT MORE STRATEGY

Perhaps we need a bit more thinking, and a bit more closed-door, behind-the-scenes scheming.

Perhaps we need to bide our time more, getting better, understanding ourselves and our businesses more instead of showcasing our every move thinking that we're being "transparent" as we pander for "likes."

Perhaps we should keep it to ourselves once in a while or, better yet, go for a long, meandering walk with a friend trying to understand the problem better.

Because solutions are impossible to find unless you define the problem. And you'll never be able to define the problem if you're dying by a thousand cuts.

CHAPTER 2

How to Succeed in Fitness Marketing Without Really Trying

"In the factory we make cosmetics; in the
drugstore we sell hope."
—*Charles Revson (founder of Revlon)*

Most fit pros waste a lot of time on their marketing. They're led astray by misguided attempts, believing that the delivery method is the most important thing.

These misinformed folk believe if a promotion fails, it's because Facebook's organic reach has gone down or there's a problem with their advertisements. Maybe these things have contributed, but they are never the root cause.

The specific marketing channel that you choose, or the specific marketing tactic you employ, matters much less than you think.

By the time a prospect is ready to buy, you should have already been developing rapport, trust, and reputation toward her for months, i.e., branding. If you've done that successfully, your marketing and advertising will profitably convert. If you don't, you could still make it happen, but it's going to be a lot harder and a lot more expensive.

What I'm about to share will feel like cheating because you'll find yourself doing less, and getting more. Before I begin, it's important to first define the difference between branding, marketing, and advertising.

People have misused and abused these terms so much that they've become meaningless. Let's establish a common definition for each:

1. **Branding** is how you go about your day. It's who you are. It's not about colors on a website or your logo. A brand is trust and reputation and expectation. It is the most valuable asset you could ever hope to attain and retain.

2. **Marketing** is the act of getting somebody to want to do what you want them to do. It is strongly rooted in psychology because, as marketing legend David Ogilvy once said, "Consumers don't think how they feel. They don't say what they think and they don't do what they say."

3. **Advertising** is also known as *direct response marketing.* It is the act of paying for attention and measuring the resulting sales. Advertising is what most fit pros consider when they think of marketing.*

While all three are separate, there's a lot of interplay between them.

If brand is strong, marketing and advertising become much easier

Not long ago, a frustrated trainer posed a question in one of our groups. Here's a snippet:

"Is it me, or are people struggling with marketing? I'm feeling like my business just can't take off and I feel so stale with it all. FB ads? Instagram? Free training? Just so muddled with it all, just makes me want to quit tbh."

Before I had a chance to answer, OTA grad Ren Jones,** owner of Fitness Jones Training, jumped in with a killer response that perfectly sums up the difference between marketing and branding ...

I appreciate there are actual defined meanings for these terms. Because they've been misused so much those terms are meaningless. We'll be using these definitions for our purposes in this book. Others may use them differently. It's kind of like the terms "metabolic" and "functional," where they once meant something and probably still do, but they've been misused so much it no longer matters.

** *Ren later became season-two host of our podcast,* It's Possible: Conversations with Successful Online Trainers. *You can listen here:* **OnlineTrainer.com/podcast.**

> *My opinion is that everyone who has challenges with branding will always have issues with marketing. Marketing is for alerting potential consumers. Reminding them you're there.*
>
> **Branding is the reason people hire us.**
> *Your personhood, so to speak. The reason I buy Nike products has much less to do with their marketing, and much more to do with their branding. They are top of mind.*
>
> *Marketing is a profile on a dating site. Branding is how the opposite sex perceives you over time.*
>
> *Branding takes time. It's what your client tells their friends about you.*

Building a business that depends on notifications is a losing proposition. That doesn't mean you should disregard them. The best way to use marketing is to, in Ren's words, "alert a potential consumer"— to let people who already see you as the expert know you sell something. Then you can pay for advertisements to convert them with a special offer.

This is how to build a robust business. It's not easy. It takes time. You'll think everybody else is doing things better and faster than you — they found a magic bullet and success comes easy.

Remember Aesop's fable The Tortoise and the Hare: "Don't brag about your lightning pace, for slow and steady won the race."

My friend Greg Nuckols, who runs Stronger by Science, summed this up in a brilliant Facebook post when he said, "If someone's really good at something, odds are pretty good that they put way more work into it than you realize, and it will take you way more work to reach their level than you'd expect."

The internet is a place where every user constantly compares his or her bloopers to others' highlight reels. The real work is always behind the scenes. No one tries to sell that because it ain't sexy. But put the right pieces in place and it'll come naturally.

Branding takes time, but the better you get at it, and the longer you work on it, the easier marketing and advertising will become.

Don't confuse the gasoline for the fire

I recently had a fun — and very telling — text exchange with OTA grad Francis McCabe, owner of Precision Online Coaching. He sent me the following:

"The guys I'm in the mastermind with can't believe how many clients I can get without a landing page or website and just closing deals with Facebook msgs lol."

Nothing about this is a surprise. It doesn't have to be Facebook, but the important stuff seems to be missed all too often in the day of the omnipresent marketing funnel that promises to somehow, magically, deliver boatloads of money ... while you sleep.

After Francis told me this, I related a story to him that I'd recently heard. Supposedly, internet personality and businessman Gary Vaynerchuk was on stage at a summit where marketers gathered to compare notes, funnels, and A/B tests. He up and called out everybody in the room by declaring, "I'm not here because of a f***ing funnel. I'm here because I'm Gary F***ing Vee."

Sounds 'bout right.

After telling him the story about Gary Vee, I get the feeling Francis is chuckling on the other side of the world. He's in Northern Ireland and a full-time firefighter who uses online training to supplement his income, commit more time to personal development, and hang with his daughter and dogs.

His response: "I like it. 1 guy who I am friendly with tried online about 2 months after me. Fancy promo video website and the lot. Well not the lot as he didn't have the results to showcase while I was doing basic Facebook posts and getting results ... he no longer does Online Coaching. He didn't invest in a course, is a PT* and just thought it would be easy. Lasted 2 months.

---

* In some places around the world, PT is a registered term for physical therapist. In other places, it's commonly used by personal trainers. In our work, because we have worldwide reach, we resist using it when speaking about trainers out of respect to physical therapists. I leave it here because this is a direct quote from Francis, who lives in Ireland where this is a commonly accepted usage.

Shocked when he realized there is no such thing as easy money ..."

Did you catch what Francis hit on there? This other guy was doing marketing and advertising but missed the part about branding. He lasted two months.

Stories like that need to be more public. Francis' friend misinterpreted the work. He got sold on a dream, built a funnel, and realized there's more to it than writing an ebook and somehow making hundreds of thousands of dollars while relaxing on a beach.

I urge you: Stop confusing the gasoline for the fire. If it was easy to set up this magical thing called a funnel that prints money, don't you think everybody would do it?

Another message from another friend popped in shortly after I went back and forth with Francis. This woman had just finished a $5,000 mentorship program and had zero ROI to show for it. What did she have? A ton of gasoline, but no fire:

- Free ebooks to give away in exchange for emails
- Meticulously edited blog content
- New format for her website
- An eight-email sequence for funneling (without anybody going into the funnel)

Remember what I said in chapter one when I quoted the *Fundamentals of Online Training* textbook: Of the thousands of people that have used this program, most have never needed to use advertising.

The reason: What I teach in OTA (and everywhere else) are fundamental principles that come first, and amplify all other efforts. They are:

- Expanding your personal network
- Relationship building
- Reputation management
- Becoming the expert

Know what else you can call those activities? BRANDING. And the results speak for themselves.

The real enemy isn't other trainers; it's Netflix

A while ago, a coach named James reached out to me:

> *"There are so many trainers on Instagram offering low-cost plans. You're telling me to charge a premium. How the heck could I compete?"*

Great question, James. Here's how I answered:

> *Being a good-enough trainer should earn you a good-enough living. But to get ahead, you need to differentiate yourself. That is, to position your products and services in a way that makes things*

easier for you.

Positioning explains why some trainers struggle for attention while others have a firehose of leads, with long waiting lists of prospects eager to pay them whatever they decide to charge.

Trainers fail because they focus on marketing, James. You need to focus on "market-making."

You fall prey to competition if you allow yourself to be compared. With that competition comes price sensitivity, which begets a race to the bottom where you'll probably lose to that bro or bro-ette on Instagram.

The real enemy isn't other trainers; it's Netflix. The real enemy is the couch. For the good of your bank account and the good of the world, we all need to fight this common enemy. Stop thinking about how you can beat other trainers, James. Make your own market by getting butts off of couches and helping people sweat and inspiring them to come back the next day for more.

James, you pull this off by fostering belief in your followers. Lucy's pulled the football away from Charlie Brown one too many times. Fitness consumers are tired of being misled. They don't believe you or anybody else, but most of all, they don't believe in themselves.

Almost everybody that you're trying to sell a transformation to has tried and failed in multiple attempts at that same transformation. Your marketing must provide hope or, better yet, a new opportunity.

Help your audience take a step in the right direction. A small, single step is all it takes. If you can help somebody take a step forward toward getting the physical transformation they desire, you've given them back the belief in themselves. With it comes a hope for a great future. Be the harbinger of that hope and you'll be the one hired to lead them the rest of the way.

It's at this point, and only this point, James, where competition becomes irrelevant from other coaches and, most of all, from Netflix. That's how you stand out, render competition irrelevant, charge what you're worth, and make an impact.

Your prospect has heard it all before and won't believe you at first.

Even if you're truly better and really can help him in ways that others cannot, you'll be ignored unless you promise something innovative. **A new mechanism or a different process represents a fresh chance at the transformation your prospect still wants, no**

matter how many times he's been disappointed.

And isn't that really what we're selling? Hope? Belief? A fresh chance? I think so.

To be clear, I'm not telling you to make anything up, embellish, or even stretch the truth. Far from it. Instead, I'm telling you to identify something exciting in the old. A new way to frame something familiar. Then make it your category of one.

Why it's about you and not all the other trainers

A good percentage of trainers go into the field because they enjoy fitness themselves, the sweating, the challenge, the drive to improve. Some got that from being athletes or former athletes. That's the mindset. And it's a good mindset, don't get me wrong. But it comes with something that can sabotage you: the need to compete.

You want to be better than everyone else on the playing field. And when you enter an industry, that's the playing field and all the other people doing what you're doing are the competition. Totally logical, totally sensible, and totally *wrong*.

The truth: If you think you're competing, you've already lost. Competition stems from incestual marketing practices. *That guy did something, he seems successful, so if I'm going to be successful, I need to do that same thing.*

Hogwash.

The easiest way to win is to play your own game. If you need competition, like I mentioned earlier, you have Netflix and the couch and everything else that pulls your clients away from your guidance and the work they need to do. Identify your position and confidently brand it as yours, independent of what else is out there. Stand out and refuse to be compared.

Is it scary? Sure. Will people say negative things about you? Yup, and you should welcome it, because that's how you know you're doing something right. Until you own your position, you can't own it in the minds of your prospects. Once you do, commit your time, money, and resources to generating interest in that market, and to reinforcing your dominant position within that market. (Another sign you're doing something right: copycats.)

Folks, this is branding. And now you can see why it's so much bigger than marketing.

Listen to Uncle Walt

Back in chapter one I mentioned one of the big blind spots for trainers: asking lousy questions. Let's revisit that for a second, because I see it in my online communities all the time and it connects to the bigger point I'll make in this section. A new coach joins and asks the same questions that have been asked over and over:

- "What's the best price to charge?"
- "How are you all getting clients?"
- "What software are you all using?"
- "What do you include in your packages?"
- "Can anybody share their online training website?"

Pay particular attention to the verbiage. Do you see a common thread?

In all cases, the questions are designed to find out *what other people are doing.*

That's human instinct. We're new to something, we're looking to learn, so the natural urge is to see what others have done, and done well. But let me tell you: The only real usefulness in finding out what others have done is strictly academic.

"But wait," you say. "Isn't it useful to learn what *doesn't* work for someone else so I can avoid it?" It can be, of course. But, what does or doesn't work for others is just information. With some work you may be able to distill some bits and pieces to apply to what you do. But it's going to mostly be a waste of your time. Why? Because two trainers could do the exact same thing and it could work brilliantly for one while the other crashes and burns.

We live in a world of infinite opportunity. I know people who are crushing it with video, paid Facebook ads, and every social media network you can think of. I also know people who are killing it with in-person networking at local Toastmasters and Chamber of Commerce events, blogging, direct mail, and local media.

Whenever a trainer asks about the best way to get clients, or tells me they're trying everything and nothing seems to work, I tell them this:

Pretty much everything works, except what you're doing.

What *can* you do? Listen to Uncle Walt.

> *"Get a good idea and stay with it. Dog it, and work at it until it's done, and done right."*
> —*Walt Disney*

Many trainers fail because they try to do too much, diluting their efforts.

Keep it simple. Choose one traffic source you can give your focus and attention to for a minimum of six months.

Which traffic source? You want the one that best suits your skillsets (that's why one strategy will work for one trainer and not another; skillsets always vary). I love to write. So I write. My YouTube account is a ghost town, I screw around on Instagram for fun, and I've never considered a personal podcast. I write, and I publish. And I do it well. And I keep getting better at it and better at selling through it.

"But Jon, people don't read anymore and Facebook says that video is more important." Whenever I'm told that "people like ___," all I want to do is look the well-intentioned advisor in the eye and ask what makes them the authority on what people like? A lot of people like a lot of different things. People who love video and hate to read don't follow me or learn from me. That's fine. They're not for me and I'm not for them.

You do you, my friend, and listen to Uncle Walt. Dog it, do it well, get better, and gradually build an audience around the traffic source that you enjoy and can continue to master. (Once again, this is all one big branding project.)

After you choose a traffic source, make it your sole focus for a minimum of six months. Learn everything you can about it and ignore all else. Develop your skillset within that medium, network in communities of others who use that traffic source, learn the ins and outs of how the platform works, and study how to convert customers using the medium.

An example:

Let's say that you love video. Cool. YouTube is going to be your thing and you may choose to syndicate to Instagram and other platforms in the future. Make it a focus, top to bottom.

- Begin shooting videos right away
- Take improv classes
- Hire a speaking coach
- Learn basic video editing

- Attend events with other YouTubers
- Study how YouTube organic discovery works
- Take note of the types of feature images, video titles, and descriptions that do well
- Do everything you can to figure out how other popular YouTubers gained their initial traction
- Learn how to convert subscribers and viewers to paying customers

Don't reinvent the wheel. Systematically break down the process and build it back up.

Go deep, not wide. Once you've implemented a single marketing plan that runs smoothly without your constant input, you can either scale up that traffic source, or systematically add new sources, one at a time.

If it really isn't working? Try something new, but don't stop. Trust me, even if the first thing doesn't work, you'll have gained invaluable insights into your brand and how people react to it. Maybe you're not unique enough? Maybe you're not a market of one? Again, none of these things happen overnight, so don't expect them to.

As you do all this, other trainers are scattered, never really getting good at anything, trying endless marketing tactics and reacting to every new possibility without ever knowing exactly what they're doing or where they're going. You, on the other hand, will be proactive. You'll know exactly what kind of business you're creating, who you're helping, why and how you serve your clients, and exactly how you'll go about getting them. You're growing your business in a strategic, stepwise fashion and developing valuable skills as you go.

The people who have the most are the people who do the basic things that you know you should do. They don't do fancy things and almost always ignore up-and-coming fads. Instead, they regularly do the boring, basic stuff that you and I both know works. This goes for business, fitness, and everything else.

DO YOU HAVE THE GUTS TO BE ... PERSISTENT?

You can try a lot of things to get your brand out there. But can you stay with it through the slowness, the times of no apparent progress, and the frustration? The real test isn't how talented a brander or marketer you are. The real test, in the esteemed words of Rocky Balboa, is how hard can you get hit and keep moving forward?

CHAPTER 3

3 Fitness Marketing Principles You Must Follow

(Ignore Them at Your Peril)

"Build something 100 people love, not something a million people kind of like."

—Brian Chesky (cofounder of Airbnb)

Now that you have a good grasp on this branding thing, we need to talk more about marketing. The entire middle section of this book is devoted to dozens of proven marketing ideas used by successful trainers. But we have some stuff to cover here first.

In this book the marketing is designed for fitness professionals and the unique business challenges we face. So anytime you hear a voice in your head piping up, "But *New York Times* bestselling author

Marketer McMarketingface says ABC is more effective for XYZ," take a breath and remember that Marketer McMarketingface isn't a fitness professional.

Lots of principles absolutely overlap. There's lots to learn from other industries. But again, right here, right now, my advice is tailored for the fit pro looking to level up.

First, we'll talk about three basic marketing principles all fit pros must follow. As you read through them, you'll also see how branding figures prominently in the conversation, like a powerline running through everything you do. That's crucial. Branding and marketing go hand in hand.

Fitness marketing principle #1: You're in the marketing business

You've heard the myth of the trainer who "just wants to help people" and "doesn't care about money." It permeates every aspect of the fitness industry and needs to stop.

You're not a volunteer. You're a professional. Professionals get paid for their work. Being passionate and helping people are not mutually exclusive.

Saying that you don't care about money is an excuse you make when you aren't confident enough to charge what you're worth. If hearing that stings, do some self-assessment because, if you're offended by it, it's probably true.

Nothing happens until you make a sale. You can't make a sale until you market your business, asking for money in exchange for the value of your services. Provide value, make money. It's that simple.

Money is an amplifier. The more money you make, the more you can do to help others. So if you want to help people. You need to make money (even if you don't care about it yourself).[*]

Whether you like it or not, you're in the marketing business. This isn't unique to fitness. Everybody who sells anything or wants to make any impact anywhere is in the marketing business.

Fitness marketing principle #2: You favor abundance over scarcity

The scarcity mindset does more damage to potentially great trainers and businesses than any other mistake. It goes like this: You're a trainer, maybe you own a gym, and you think highly of your talents to the point where you don't want to share anything you know or do. Your

---

[*] *I'm an example of somebody who doesn't particularly care about money. Or, more specifically, fancy things. By choice, I drive a 12-year-old car with 200,000 kilometers on it, I don't own a watch, and all of my favorite pastimes are free (hiking, biking, being with family). That said, I'm acutely aware the more money the company makes, the more amazing things we can produce and the more impact we have. I make millions not because I care about personally having millions. I do it because I know it's the only way to help more people.*

"trade secrets" are sacred. There's only so much to go around and your share of the market is always ripe for poaching.

The fitness business is about community. Cross-pollination across communities, working together, and forging profitable partnerships, is the best thing we can do to help our businesses win. That, and what you know probably isn't that much of a secret anyway ...

Leave the scarcity mindset behind. Embrace abundance and let it show and flow through all your branding and marketing. The fitness industry is *massive*. There's ample business for everybody. Take your fair share, but don't forget to share what you take.

Those who act abundantly, support others, give without any thought of what they'll get in return, and don't keep score soon realize what they get back is worth many times more.

Fitness marketing principle #3: You believe in attracting customers to you

The most successful trainers have prospects seeking them out. They practice "attraction marketing." You may have heard the term before — it's not new.

The concept is simple: You brand and market yourself in a way that makes you the obvious choice for prospects. You establish yourself as an expert within your prospects' community. You do a great job and make sure everyone knows it. You treat your clients like all-stars. Your reputation precedes you.

This takes time, obviously. And yes, you'll do some selling and following up with prospects as you build your brand and rep. But attraction is one of your marketing goals. You want people coming to you with money in their hands, asking you how to buy, happy to pay whatever you charge.

MARKETING IS ADDING VALUE, NOT TRICKERY

Marketing doesn't mean manipulating people into doing things they don't want to do.

Ethical marketing is simply identifying a need and figuring out ways to make yourself the go-to for that need, for as long as you need to, until somebody decides that they want to hire a trainer. When that happens, you'll have already positioned yourself as the obvious choice.

So ... are you marketing yourself yet?

Something you may not know but need to understand: Methods and tools change, but why humans buy remains the same and purchase decisions are rarely based on merit.

Yes, in some cases, consumers try to educate

themselves on a product and sales outlet (car shopping, for example), but by and large, consumers make terrible, uninformed purchase decisions that have little to do with good reasons. They rely on cues from others and representative info that allows them to justify their purchase decision.

I hit on this in chapter one and want to revisit it here in more detail, because you've done this and I've done this.

Near the beginning of the book I talked about wanting to buy a TV with moving pictures. I like that example because it happened to me, and the salesperson was smart enough to give me a reason to purchase, right then and there.

Years ago, my roommate moved out and took his TV with him. I needed a new TV. Now, I don't know anything about TVs, so I walked into the first electronic store I could find and browsed. They had rows and rows of TVs — at least 50. I'd have been happy with just about any one of them. All I needed was something that had moving pictures.

Enter the salesperson.

He asked me what I wanted to watch. I said sports. He told me to get a TV with a good "Hertz Rate" because it makes fast moving images crisper.*

I bought the TV with a good Hertz Rate.

I had no idea what Hertz Rate was before I walked into the store, aside from the obvious rental car confusion. I *still* don't know what it is. He might have made it up — I never checked (and please don't ever tell me if you bump into me, I don't want to know). I had no idea whether the image was crisper and I didn't care. I was happy with the TV. It had color and moving pictures. This was all I wanted anyway.

I, the ignorant consumer, wanted an excuse to make a decision. The salesman gave me one. I was there because I wanted a TV. Not selling me a TV would have been a disservice to me.

Yet, if he'd made it more complicated by asking me more technical questions, I wouldn't have felt confident buying the TV that day. I'd have said I needed to "think about it" because I wouldn't have wanted to lose face in front of the TV expert by showing him my ignorance. I'd have wanted to go home and educate myself more. When all I wanted the entire time was a box that let me

---

* *Recall idiosyncratic fit heuristic from chapter one (if this is you, then this is for you).*

The salesman asked one question to figure out who I was (that I wanted to watch sports) and immediately followed with a recommendation for a TV that was right "for me." That's all it took, and often all it takes.

watch the Toronto Maple Leafs lose yet another game.*

Now apply this to your business. In almost every case when somebody shops for a fitness coach or program, this is the process:

- She has a problem. It's painful (this can be psychological pain, as with being overweight).
- She's had this problem before, or it's never gone away.
- She hasn't been able to solve this problem after repeated attempts.
- She wants the problem to go away as quickly and easily as possible.
- She doesn't know how to solve the problem, and it feels like it's impossible to figure out the right steps.
- This sucks, and feels like it's always going to suck.

What happens next depends on how you've branded and marketed yourself.

The chances that this prospect stands before you by some random alignment of the stars is low. Sure, maybe she simply walked into the gym where you work and you happened to be standing near the front desk. But more likely, she's talking to you because something you did previously to establish your worth caught her eye.

---

* *If you ever want to study self-loathing and get a feel for what decades of disappointment and frustration feel like, come to Toronto and speak to a few hockey fans.*

Maybe her cousin referred you. Maybe your niche matches up with her goal and you're the leading name in that niche. It could be a dozen possibilities. The point is, she found you and wants to talk.

Guess what? If you've properly branded and marketed yourself, you won't have to depend on your personal equivalent of Hertz Rate to get her to buy. Her purchase rationale is already in place. She's convinced you're the one. You won't complicate things. You won't give her an excuse to "think it over." You'll reinforce her confidence in her purchase, even if she's not sure why you're the ideal choice beyond what she knows about you (true customer satisfaction comes later when you give her great results).

Scenarios like this are why I stress the following: Don't wait. Dig the well before you're thirsty. Get ahead of it and make your market.

Build your communities. Develop your reputation. Control your fate. And keep it simple.

How to hire your professor

Years ago, I had a long dinner conversation with a highly successful investment advisor, someone who manages more than $1 billion for his clients. Before he became that, he paid his way through school as a photographer. He was so good at business, in fact, that he hired his photography professor to develop film for him on weekends.

How you react to that last sentence says a lot about how you see the world.

Most people would think the circumstances should be the opposite. The professor should be the one who employs the student. Isn't he the one with the superior knowledge?

Maybe. But that's not how the world works.

The job doesn't require advanced knowledge. Like fitness, a decent photographer is good enough for 99 percent of the people who hire photographers. In my friend's case, the main business was taking sorority and fraternity headshots ... not exactly complicated stuff.

The prof, we can guess, made barely enough to get by. But his student, who knew less about photography, nonetheless managed to hustle up so much work that he had to pay someone to help him. The teacher needed money, the student needed help, and the unusual arrangement worked out fine for both of them.

In our industry, we often see the most knowledgeable trainers get frustrated and burned out. They work long hours and do great work for their clients, but they never seem to get ahead because their work has become commoditized.

What most clients need is way less than the advanced expertise this trainer has attained over the years. And instead of learning the littlest bit about business and branding and marketing, the fit pro instead delves deeper into training. It is, after all, more comfortable to learn more about a topic you're already an expert in than to acquire a new skill.

The trainer burns out because she reaches the top of the pay scale for what she does in the company. And who sets that scale? Probably someone who knows less than she does.

Too often, I hear fitness pros say things like, "My programs are great. People should buy from me, and not from that guy on Instagram," or, "I've been working so hard for so many years, I should be getting paid more."

Forget "should." Strike it from your vocabulary. How things should be is irrelevant. What matters is how they are. If the system doesn't work for you, you can either work to change it, find a way to get around it, or invent a better system, one that works to your advantage.

THROUGHOUT HISTORY, THE WEALTHIEST PEOPLE HAVE NEVER BEEN THE SMARTEST.

They've been the most resourceful. Society's value system doesn't reward the people who get results. *It rewards the people who get credit for the results.* There's a big difference.

CHAPTER 4

7 Components of Compelling Offers That Leave Clients Begging to Buy

"Personally, I am very fond of strawberries and cream, but I have found that for some strange reason, fish prefer worms."

—Dale Carnegie

A compelling offer has seven components, which I'll get into in a moment. First, I'd like to talk to you about your prices. More specifically, raising them.

For many fit pros, your first step is often to raise your prices. It doesn't *have* to be, but almost every fitness pro whose services are in demand could charge more.*

Let's say you raise your prices by 30 percent. You won't lose 30 percent of your customers, but you may find yourself working fewer hours and making more money. For most trainers, it's the fastest, easiest win.

The next step is to invest your newfound time and capital on something that helps your business grow even more — hiring contract help, developing marketing systems, or creating a product or intellectual property that, in turn, gives you even more time and more money. When you reinvest that time and those funds, the cycle speeds up.

The specifics vary from person to person, but whatever they're doing tends to follow a pattern: To create more value and revenue, you need to stop selling time and start selling transformation. The easiest way to sell transformations is to craft what marketing expert Dan Kennedy calls a *compelling offer*.

The more compelling the offer, the easier it'll be to market and sell. A compelling offer has the following seven components (this list comes directly from Kennedy with application to the fitness industry from me):

---

* *Pricing is a separate and complicated subject, but some people get very weird when it's time to talk money. I've seen charismatic, likable pros get shy and hesitant when it's time to talk money. My advice: Get over it.*

Money is the entire point of being a professional trainer. It's your business. It's your food and shelter, and your future. It's your ability to elicit even more change. I'd prefer trainers get so confident about "time to talk money" that it's the most exciting part of the process for them.

The 7 Steps to a Compelling Offer

1. A clear, specific promise.
2. A specific deadline (generally 90 days or less).
3. A strong value proposition.
4. A reward for immediate action (scarcity).
5. Asking for the sale.
6. A powerful guarantee.
7. A specific leader.

Here's a bit more on each:

1. A clear, specific promise.

As Kennedy says, "Confused people don't buy." The more clear you are in your marketing materials about who your program is for, and what they'll get, the easier it will be to sell.

I see a lot of marketing break down not when it says too little, but when it says too much. You can have multiple programs for different prospects, but you can't sell to any of them until you know the desired result for each customer.

2. A specific deadline (generally 90 days or less).

We all know a healthy lifestyle has no deadline. You shouldn't stop exercising or eating well after three months. But when you sell a transformation, there must be an end in sight.

Anything longer than 90 days for a new client is

generally too intimidating (or worse, too labor-intensive). Your clients want to know how long the magic will take, so meet them at a defined endpoint. Once you help them get started, you've earned the buy-in to help them stick with the program long enough for it to become a lifestyle.

3. A strong value proposition.

What does your customer value? Time, money, flexibility, hard work, or something else? You'll find out in your initial conversations with a prospect. It could be different for each one. Whatever it is, make it the major selling point for your program.

4. A reward for immediate action (scarcity).

You must give a client a reason to hand over his credit card and act now. Here's how you create a sense of scarcity,* taken directly from the Online Trainer Academy textbook, *The Fundamentals of Online Training*. Keep in mind you can mix and match:

> Limited-time offer. *Clients must register before a set date. After that, they'll either miss out completely or be forced to wait a long time for another chance.*

---

* *Don't confuse this definition of scarcity with "scarcity mindset," which I warned against in chapter three. That was based on selfishness and standoffishness. Here I'm talking about products/services that appear special, desirable, and urgent because either people can't get them anywhere else or they won't be available after a certain deadline.*

Limited-time bonus. *Clients can still register after a set date, but they won't get the awesome bonus early birds get, which could be anything from a free month of training to an ebook, water bottle, or T-shirt.*

Price increase. *Clients who register after a set date have to pay more than those who act sooner.*

5. Asking for the sale.

Again, money makes some people weird. If you want somebody to give you money, you have to ask for it. Sounds obvious, but most fitness pros should do it more often.

6. A powerful guarantee.

A guarantee can convert more sales than almost any other aspect of your marketing. A guarantee reverses the risk, making the purchase a no-brainer by reinforcing the value proposition. If the client doesn't get the promised results, you don't get her money. For example, if your 90-day transformation program guarantees a loss of three inches, the guarantee could say "three inches down or your money back."

The best guarantees reinforce the value proposition. If clients value their time, you guarantee that you won't waste it and that you won't be late to a session. If they value a specific type of result, then you guarantee results. Most guarantees that you see are money-back guarantees and these aren't bad, but they are often considerably less effective than guaranteeing your value proposition.

7. A *specific leader.*

Every community needs a leader. The leader is the expert. This doesn't mean the leader needs to be out front offering the deliverables day in and day out, but she does need to be the face and voice of the operation.

CLOSING PART ONE: THE JOY OF A BAD PLAN

A while back, my friend wanted to learn guitar. He wanted to do it right, so he did his research. He spent time on forums, asked people he knew about the "best way," and studied what all of the experts suggested as the best way to learn.

Six months passed. My friend had yet to pick up a guitar. When he told me this story he added, "If I had gone to the closest guitar shop, bought the cheapest guitar, watched a few YouTube videos, and started plugging away, I'd be six months ahead of where I am today."

I know that we've covered a lot thus far and it might seem like there's a lot you have to do before getting started. Please don't interpret it that way. You don't have to nail every point in this book. You won't anyway even if you try.

Sometimes all you need is to go to the closest store, buy the cheapest guitar, and start plugging away. You'll likely be lacking a clear plan and you certainly won't have a good plan. Heck, it might even be a bad plan.

But a bad plan successfully implemented will lead to mistakes, which will teach you lessons, which will lead to improvement.

So my advice to you as we round out part one and prepare to indulge into the main part of this book is to make a bad plan. A bad plan is better than no plan. A bad plan is a good start.

PART TWO

50 Proven Ways to Get More Clients

Special Introduction to This Section

This section is devoted to specific, strategic methods for getting more clients.

The ideas are diverse and come from a diverse group of fitness experts — we'll shout out those names where appropriate — who have become incredibly successful by doing one thing really well.

But first I wanted to take a moment and explain how I've organized them.

This section contains three chapters, each packed with tips and advice under a separate heading to help you see how they function best.

(Oh, and even though I say there are "50 ways" in this section, that's just the numbered subjects we talk about. The real number, with tips and sub-tips and other pearls within those subjects, is easily in the hundreds.)

Chapter five collects some incredibly valuable **long-term strategies**, things you do consistently that tee you up for success or you put into place once and leave alone. They're important, but aren't designed to convert prospects right away.

Chapter six is all about **one-off promotions**. Smart trainers always have something new and exciting going on; here's where you'll find those ideas. Pick what feels best for your situation and crush it.

Chapter seven covers one of my favorite activities: **guerrilla marketing**. All I can say is: Respect the importance of always being ready...

CHAPTER 5

Savvy Long-Term Client Conversion Strategies

"Dig the well before you are thirsty."

—Chinese Proverb

The most successful trainers think long-term and apply as many of the savvy strategies you're about to learn consistently over months and years.

Kicking off part two are a series of seriously underrated yet important techniques for getting clients. What follows is not sexy and will not bring you instant gratification.

These strategies are basically, "Here's what the most successful people do behind the scenes that's really led to their success that nobody talks about or sees."

These strategies are the seeds you plant so that you

wake up a year later in a position where business generates itself.

1. Getting testimonials in a non-awkward way you can actually use

Every trainer should have a collection of testimonials from past and current clients.

In an industry rife with dishonesty and associated distrust, it's important for you to add in as many proof elements as possible before making a sales proposition. Getting testimonials* for personal training is the best way to do it.

For gym owners or salespeople, imagine the power of having a full binder sitting in the reception area for potential clients to flip through as they wait for a tour, complimentary session, or sales meeting. For online trainers, imagine a testimonial page on your website brimming with inspiring stories and before/after photos.

A great testimonial is not a client saying, "Oh, I love Jon, he's awesome." A useful testimonial consists of one ideal client saying things that will resonate with another *potential* ideal client (remember, I touched on identifying your ideal client in chapter two).

---

* Testimonials aren't quite the same as referrals, which you'll hear a lot more about in part three of this book, but they are cousins. Once you read about referral culture in chapters eight and nine, you'll see how it all works together.

If you're just starting out, I suggest creating fictional avatars of your "ideal" client types and then using that information to inform how and what you'll ask for in a testimonial. For example, one might read like so:

> *A 26-year-old woman who is 30 pounds overweight. She's never used a trainer and is finally looking for some direction after numerous failed attempts at the gym. She's nervous and shy and uncomfortable in the gym, and this has always turned her off training. Additionally, she's a nurse, so shift work makes regular sleep and food habits hard to come by.*

I suggest you create three or four ideal client avatars in a similar fashion (but with much more detail). This way you'll know what aspects of the testimonial you want to highlight with prospects who have similar goals and limitations.

Here's an example of a strong testimonial that would be perfect to show my made-up client above:

> *I wasn't obese when I started to train with Jon, but definitely had some weight to lose. It's funny, you know, I'd been in the gym on and off for a few years without much to show for it. I didn't believe a trainer would really be able to help me until I had "worked my way up to it." I've been in gyms before and, to be honest, felt judged and uncomfortable so I never considered working*

*with trainers who seemed like they were from
another planet. I also work shifts — sometimes
nights — and don't sleep well.*

*What I particularly liked about Jon was how
down to earth he was. He didn't pressure me and
I felt like he really, deeply, wanted to help me
however best he could from the moment that we
met.*

*He looked at me as a whole, as opposed to giving
me some exercises and counting the sets and
reps. It took a bit of time, but he first helped me
establish better sleep habits. Jon also took a look
at what I ate and helped me identify what foods I
really loved, and which ones I could live without.
I still got to indulge but got rid of empty calories
that I didn't even enjoy. It's crazy how many
calories are in everyday foods that can easily be
replaced!*

*It didn't take long to lose a few pounds with a
couple quick changes to my diet. That got me
hooked and, six months later, not only am I at
my target weight (30 lbs down) but I didn't
suffer and I can maintain this while still living
the life I want to live. It's really amazing. I'd
recommend Jon to anybody!*

With this story, selling a client would be pretty easy, don't you think?

The above example client and testimonial are made-up, but meant to showcase how important it is to have testimonials specific to your avatar. Notice how my testimonial shows how all major reservations have been solved with my training?

In order to gather high-quality client testimonials, institute a periodic review system of your services. There are four reasons to ask for reviews and not testimonials:

1. It's much less awkward and you can ask multiple times over the time a client trains with you, thereby giving you more material to potentially use.
2. It allows you to gather much deeper material to turn into a story that can act as a powerful marketing piece.
3. It's easier for the client.
4. It may help you get better.

Here's how it works: Once a client starts training with you, schedule a review every two to three months (so you don't need to think about it). Whenever you get a calendar reminder, hand your client the review form.

Keep the review form itself short and sweet. Begin with the three *start, stop, keep* questions taken from Scott Stratten's book *UnMarketing* and follow with a few quick bits to round out the story.

You can either create a simple document, print it, and hand it to your client or use an online form. Here's what it might look like with eight sample questions to use already filled in.

YOUR BUSINESS NAME/LOGO HERE

Note: This is meant for information purposes only. J. Goodman Consulting Inc. will hold no legal responsibility if you choose to use this for your own business.

1. What's one thing that you'd like me to start doing?

2. What's one thing that you'd like me to stop doing?

3. What's one thing that you'd like me to keep doing?

4. In three sentences or less, can you describe any reservations that you had before we started working together?

5. In three sentences or less, can you explain how I was able to help you with your reservations?

6. Can you describe one or two top goals when you started?

7. In point form, please list your achievements with training thus far.

8. Is there anything else you'd like to add?

A sample review form you're welcome to use to get feedback and ultimately turn into an ongoing testimonial generation tool.

Ask every client to review you every two to three months. All you need to say is, "It's review time again" and hand them the sheet. Not everybody will return it. But most will. Sometimes you'll get great info to use, and sometimes not. Obviously the more you get, the better, but you really only need a few stories like this.

Once you get the form back, look it over to see whether it can be turned into a testimonial. If so, take the info on it and move things around into something like the example I shared earlier that you can use. Tell the best story you can.

Then, once done, message the client and first thank her for filling out your review and then tell her you took the liberty of rewriting it into a review for your services. Send her the text and ask if it's okay to use it for promotional purposes. Once she says yes, you're good to go.*

2. A simple way to create goodwill, show how much you care, and close clients

*From Pete Dupuis, vice president and business director of Cressey Sports Performance (**petedupuis.com**)*

---

* *Whenever using before-and-after photos, testimonials like this, or similar materials, always get permission from the client. This can be done either when she starts by having her sign off that her photos may be used for promotional purposes in perpetuity moving forward or whenever you ask. Then keep a folder backed up on your computer called "permissions" where you store the email or scans of paper she signed off on. Odds that anybody will ever get angry or, in the worst-case scenario, file a lawsuit against you, are slim to none. But this is still a good idea.*

Winter is the busiest time of the year at Cressey Sports Performance (CSP), where we train baseball players getting ready for the upcoming season. This is when we show how much we know. We do it partially by asking the right questions and making the right adjustments to their programs. But mostly we showcase our knowledge the way all trainers do: by making our athletes stronger, faster, and more impervious to injury.

Once the season starts, though, we show how much we care. We pay our staff to get to as many games as possible — high school and college games in the spring; travel, amateur, and minor-league games in the summer.

It would be easy to track these guys on social media, giving them shout-outs on Twitter and Instagram. But it's far more effective to show up in person, to shake hands with the parents and make small talk in the stands.

By stepping outside of our comfort zone, we create goodwill with our existing clients while also attracting new ones:

- Our athletes get to engage with us on their turf, instead of inside the gym, where we call the shots.

- The parents who pay us to train their kids are genuinely thrilled to see us. It shows we care about them not just as clients, but as athletes and people.

- Those parents sing our praises as they introduce us to other parents. You think it's great when a client introduces you to a prospect via email? Wait until you're introduced to a group of dads as "the trainer I've been telling you all about."

- You know who's not at the games? Our competition. Parents looking at our websites may not be able to tell which facility would be better for their kids. But when we show up and the other guys don't (we wear CSP T-shirts, so it's easy to pick us out in a crowd), we make their decision a lot easier.

Don't train athletes? You still have lots of ways to show you care about your clients. They're all passionate about things outside the gym. Your job is to identify those interests, and figure out how to show your support. In my decade as a gym owner I've shown up for garage band performances, sat through less-than-impressive stand-up comedy routines, and accepted invitations to graduation parties made up almost entirely of close friends and family members.

For you it might be baby showers and birthday parties if you work with pregnant or postnatal women, or charity events for more affluent clients. Whatever it is, this simple gesture goes a long way.

3. Win awards and leverage the unprecedented social proof that follows

*From Lisa Simone Richards, public relations and visibility strategist for health and fitness entrepreneurs (**lisasimonerichards.com**)*

You'll read a lot in this book about becoming that go-to fit pro for people, about becoming the best in their eyes and generating irresistible word-of-mouth and referrals.

If you really have the skills and reputation, why not get some third-party recognition for it you can then use when you try all the other ideas in this book? And even if a potential client has heard of you, how do they know the difference between #1 and #10 in your area? That's where awards come in.

When I worked for a company that specialized in women-only bootcamps, we set out to collect as many awards as we could. It was a key marketing strategy for us, and we won them year after year in both fitness and business categories, including awards for best gym and best small or medium employer. We also got listed among hot new growth companies and top companies run by women.

The impact was huge. In just a few years we went from 30 locations across Canada to more than 100. Our annual revenues increased tenfold to $4 million. We regularly sold out sessions weeks in advance, while other bootcamps targeting our female audience struggled to reach 50 percent capacity.

Once we were the undisputed best operation in our category, we didn't need to make extraordinary efforts to attract clients. The recognition from third parties spoke for itself.

How do you win awards? Apply for them. Just about

every town, big or small, has some outlet that gives away annual "Best of ..." awards. It might be a daily or weekly paper, a city or regional magazine, a radio or TV station, or a popular local website. The voters might be readers, viewers, local experts, or the editors themselves. No matter who decides, these awards carry weight with consumers and create prestige for your brand.

Some categories, like Best Boutique Fitness Studio or Best Personal Trainer, are obvious targets. But you can also put your name in the mix for something like Top 30 Entrepreneurs Under 30, or nominate your gym for Best Places to Work.

So pay attention to local award timetables and marshal your support accordingly. And here's one last trick: *Ask the host to create a new award.* If you have a popular group class, for example, and there's no award for that, you can suggest they add Best Bootcamp or Best Spin Class. Better still, have your supporters do it for you.

The best part? Once you win, you're always a winner in your promotional materials and can include mention of it in everything you do moving forward.

4. Actually convert your free consults with these key strategies

*From Tim Henriques, director of the National Personal Training Institute (**nationalpti.org**)*

Free consults can be a huge part of building your business, and offering some combination of complimentary goal-setting session or workout can help land clients.

But it's risky. You waste valuable time and effort on every freebie that doesn't convert. Focusing on these key areas, you can drastically improve your closing ratio on new prospects:

— **Call the client the night before the session.** This serves both as a reminder for the client to show up for the session and to see if this person is truly interested in your service. My own closing percentage *doubled* after I started calling clients the night before the first session.

When you contact your client, don't text. You want to engage and start building rapport. Call the client at a reasonable hour (4 to 8 p.m. works well), introduce yourself, explain why you're calling, and answer any questions they may have. Be friendly, but succinct. If the client starts to bombard you with detailed questions that require detailed answers, politely remind him to ask those questions during training, as that's part of its purpose. Wrap it up by telling him to be ready for a fun workout, and you'll take care of everything else.

You might lose a few people right then and there, but that's okay. They probably weren't interested in the first place. I'd rather find that out over the phone in five minutes than after a full hour the next day.

GATHER THE RIGHT INFORMATION BEFORE A FREE WORKOUT

From Pat Koch, a Boston-based fitness manager and sports nutritionist

The number-one mistake you can make with a free workout is diving right into the workout. Take some time to sit down with your prospect to get to know him. Ask friendly, but targeted questions. Connect with him. Yes, medical history, injuries, and fitness level are important, but go deeper than that. Ask questions like:

> *"What do you want your body to look like?"*

> *"What's been stopping you from reaching your goals?"*

Best case: Your prospect admits something he wouldn't admit to a friend. If you can reach that level of rapport, you've clearly gained his trust.

— **Bring the serious fun**. Turn up your energy and "fun factor" during the complimentary session. This is your chance to show what it'll be like to work with you. It doesn't have to be all fun and games. If the prospect has a specific goal in mind, give him a sampling of what it'll take to get there (remember, most commercial gym members are looking for fat loss, so you'd be foolish to fixate on other areas unless the client asks). It could be simply showing the client a new exercise, a new stretching technique, or simply helping him complete his first successful workout.

— **Introduce the prospect to at least three people in the gym during the first session.** Gyms are very intimidating for many people. Treat the new client like a guest in your home and introduce him to your friends, coworkers, and other gym members to break down his walls and stereotypes about the gym and help him be more comfortable.

Knowing names and faces also helps your client feel more like he belongs, like he could really see himself working out and spending time there. You might want to give your coworkers a heads-up that you will be doing this so they know to be extra friendly.

— **Ask "yes" questions.** At the end of the session, I want you to ask the client: "Was that workout fun for you?" And he'd better say "yes." The point here is to make sure the complimentary session doesn't give your client the impression that training with you will be torture (unless that's the kind of motivation he wants).

Most people don't find throwing up, almost blacking out, and/or crying fun, so the client should not do any of those things in the first session (or at any time during training, ideally). His "yes" is affirmation for himself as well and can have an impact on the final sale.

Some other good questions include:

Do you think that workout would help you achieve your goals?

Could you do that workout two or three times a week?

You ask a question; they say "yes" in response. The point of these "yes" questions is making the prospect confirm over and over again that he does want to be in better shape; he does want to improve his health; he does need help constructing workouts and nutrition plans; and he does need a personal trainer — you. When it comes time to purchase personal training sessions, he's already primed to say "yes."

5. Offer a great guarantee

A strong guarantee is a powerful route to more sales. A guarantee inspires trust. It shows you believe in your product and are willing to stand behind it. In our sales training at the Online Trainer Academy, we teach our students to future-pace three months ahead by asking:

"If we were meeting here three months from today, what needs to have happened for you to feel happy about your progress?"

No matter how she answers, imagine how she'll react if you ask this follow-up:

"What would it mean to you if I guaranteed you'll be successful?"

Now you've not only gotten the prospect to visualize her own transformation, you've given her certainty it will happen. Because you don't get paid if it doesn't happen.

A strong guarantee ...

... uses strong language like "unconditional," "100 percent satisfaction guaranteed," "iron-clad," and "no questions asked."

... is visible. Make it a key element of promotional materials.

... asks for the sale. "Register and pay for your training today and work with us for 90 days. If we don't notice transformational results after that time, we'll refund 100 percent of your money."

Hint: "Transformational" results should be measured, so assess your client on day one for things like strength, cardio fitness, and movement capacity (mobility and flexibility) that can show provable results after a certain time.

You can guarantee three things, separately or together:

1. Product
2. Service
3. Results

A product guarantee is the most common. It sounds something like this:

> *"If you're not completely satisfied with our service, let us know and we'll return 100 percent of your money within X days."*

A service guarantee is more common for fit pros because it shows a commitment to providing time, attention, and expertise — a trainer's three most valuable commodities. It might look like this:

> *"We've attained the top certifications and qualifications available in the fitness industry to make sure you get the best experience possible. You won't find better trainers, or trainers who care more about you. But if you do, we'll refund 100 percent of your training fees."*

Or this:

> *"Your time is valuable. I guarantee I'll make every second count. When we're together, you're my only focus, and I'll always be prepared and ready for you, from the first minute of our sessions to the last. In addition, I promise to:*
>
> - *Invest as much time as needed to understand your unique life, time restraints, and nutrition challenges.*
>
> - *Work in conjunction with any other health professionals you're currently seeing*

> *(including but not exclusive to physicians,*
> *physical therapists, and massage therapists)*
> *to ensure you get effective and well-rounded*
> *care.*
>
> - *Utilize my extensive experience with strength*
>   *training, calisthenics, gymnastics, and*
>   *movement techniques to deliver pain-free*
>   *results.*
>
> - *Custom-design a personal training*
>   *experience that's perfect for you."*

A results guarantee looks something like this:

> *"Halevy Life is the world's only gym to ensure*
> *your fitness investment with a money-back*
> *guarantee. Give us 90 days and we will*
> *transform you. And we're so sure of it that at*
> *the end of 90 days, if you haven't improved in at*
> *least* three of five *quantifiable fitness measures,*
> *we'll simply return your money and cancel your*
> *membership."**

A strong guarantee makes it easier to sell at higher
price points. Occasionally a bad egg will take advantage
but these are few and far between. The benefits of
a sensational guarantee far outweigh the potential

---

* *This is a real guarantee that garnered national attention in 2015 by*
Halevy Life, a gym in New York City. An article published by Inc.com
called it "probably the craziest (and smartest) money-back guarantee
ever."

drawbacks. If you're confident in your business and service, offer an unparalleled guarantee.

6. Have (even the smallest) web presence

You don't need a big, expensive website (but it wouldn't hurt). You don't even need a medium-grade, medium-priced website (still wouldn't hurt). But you do need some kind of web presence that presents your best face and reputation to the world. If necessary, set up a free site at about.me while you plan and save for Your Website 2.0. Just have *something* people can see. People will Google you before they reach out. You never know how many potential clients you're losing by not being able to be found online.

7. Master everyday "prospecting"

*From Jennette Holzworth, owner of 5:17 Total Body Transformations (**517transformed.com**)*

It was 82 degrees Fahrenheit in the middle of a Northern California drought, yet there I was, dressed in black from head to toe — in a polo shirt no less — chasing my toddler around the playground. My friend thought I was crazy, in disbelief that using my prospecting technique during our playdate would yield any results.

She was pleasantly surprised when I walked away with a new client. But for this working mom who'd recently moved her in-home training practice to a new city, playdates and shopping trips aren't what they seem. They're an opportunity to network with potential clients and establish myself in a new community.

I specialize in women's health and fitness training, with a particular focus on family nutrition and wellness. A fenced-in toddler play yard is the barrel for my proverbial fish, and the uniform is the harpoon that reels them in. I don't have to do anything other than be myself.

I don't have to reach out and ask if someone's looking for a trainer, which can get awkward. If another mom is in the market, she will bring up the subject. If not, it's still known what I'm about and she will tell her friends about the trainer mom she met at the playground.

You are your own walking billboard, rent free!

You are your own walking billboard, rent free!

And what cheaper way to prospect than by being friendly? I would never in a million years be able to penetrate this market if I spent my time handing out pamphlets and solicitation requests to moms juggling toddlers. Instead, I'm able to start with my best foot forward — a smile, warm greeting, and conversations about temper tantrums. The rest just falls into place.

The playground might not be the best place for you to lurk when prospecting new clients, especially if you don't have a child. Instead, visit a coffeehouse (more on this in the guerrilla marketing chapter), sports shop, or other venue where your prospective clients frequent.

Without getting weird or forceful, strike up conversations about anything other than personal training and let things flow. It doesn't have to be complex or scripted; in fact, the more natural and genuine, the better. A simple smile and hello is an easy segue into a chat about the weather, extra-long lines, or last night's game.

No one wants to be sold, or preached at, but almost everyone loves making new friends. Make that your focus and business will pour in.

8. Build a client army

People always ask me, "Jon, how did you get clients when you were a trainer?" Know what? I never made flyers, gave free workshops at local businesses, canvassed the streets, or made endless cold calls to get more clients. I've also never made a hard sell in my life. None of these things are inherently bad, but most trainers worth their salt never need to use them to build up their own clientele.

People used to come to me asking to train. After

my first six to eight months, my clientele was 100 percent referral-based and I was so busy that I earned commissions from referring my overload of clients to other trainers.

Why? Because my clients became my army. The best example is a woman named Pam.

Pam had been training with me for six months when my club opened its second location. I elected to move locations. Pam was 67 years old when she started at our gym and had never worked out before.

Imagine how daunting a task it was for Pam to join the gym. She later told me that she was shaking the day we first met.

I took care of Pam from day one. All these years later, she's still working out.

The early days of her training were more classroom than workout. I taught her jargon, introduced her to everybody (staff and clientele), and did everything in my power to make her feel comfortable.*

The result? Pam almost single-handedly filled my schedule in the new location.

At one point, I was training Pam, her best friend, her

---

*An example: I called the deadlift "broom bum" (because she started with a dowel) to make it more comfortable when starting out. For six years, the exercise was called broom bum — even when Pam broom-bummed 95 pounds for a clean six reps at 70 years old. What started as a way to make her comfortable became our little thing, and little things like this are what make the trainer-client dynamic so special.

best friend's friend, her husband, her daughter, her daughter's husband, her daughter's best friend, and her daughter's best friend's friend.

In a week: 16 training hours × $41.80/hour = $668.80
In a month: 16 hours × 4 weeks = 64 hours × $41.80/hour = $2,675.20
In a year: 64 hours × 12 months = 768 hours × $41.80/hour = $32,102.40

$32,102.40. I'd say making Pam comfortable in the gym paid off. Pam was easily responsible for over $100,000 in training revenues for me by the time that I left training in 2012 to focus on building the Personal Trainer Development Center full time. Since then, she's been responsible for $100,000 in two other trainers' pockets as well (you're welcome, guys).

Here's a breakdown:

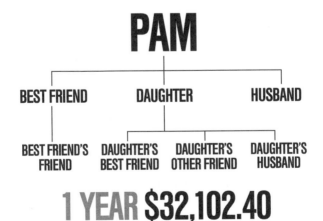

Not every client has the potential to be a Pam, but some do. You can't have my Pam, but here are a few ways to get your own:

— *Teach workout jargon.* Introduce your clients to the workout culture. Tell them what a set, rep, hypertrophy, and even RDL mean. Make sure that they know why they're doing an exercise and what energy system they're developing.

Your clients want to show off their knowledge. They want the opportunity to tell their friends and family that they performed two sets of eight reps of the deadlift (or broom bum).

The other great benefit is feeling a connection to the culture. Retention will increase and relapse into inactivity will go down.

— *Introduce them to everybody.* This is a great first-day strategy, but you should never stop. Your clients should be the most popular people in the gym. It's to your benefit that they know and are comfortable speaking to everybody. Because, guess what? If they feel popular they'll chat up new members. Guess who they'll be chatting about?

Introduce them to all the staff and members. I even went for occasional post-workout walks with my clients to get coffee in the neighborhood where our gym was located and went out of my way to introduce them to all the local shop owners.*

If your client knows everybody in the gym, they will stay longer. It becomes a social atmosphere and comfortable haven from their crazy lives that they look forward to.

— *Surprise them with emails.* Keep in touch with your clients outside of the session. You can do this via sending jokes, relevant info, restaurant advice, etc.

Back when I was shadowing trainers, helping them get better, I'd notice that many of them were only doing half the battle. While speaking with a client, they'd get an idea to send them a relevant article. The mistake? They'd tell their client about it.

When you get an idea to send a client a relevant article or joke (or just about anything), make a note on your clipboard and continue the workout. Later that evening or the next day, send them an email without notice with the subject line: *I thought you would enjoy this.*

The surprise effect keeps you in your clients' minds even on off days. It shows you're thinking of them outside of training. You know you've done well when they send you funny jokes, restaurant advice, relevant articles, etc., on *their* off days.

— *Make up your own award.* Back in the day I designed

---

* *Doing these things every day is a hallmark of an effective trainer. It's a good example of a time and place where the stuff not taught in books (until now) is more important than the stuff that is.*

a monthly award for my clients. It was called the HAF badge (HAF = Hard As F**k). In addition to getting the physical badge to display I profiled the client in a write-up on my site highlighting their accomplishments. You better believe it lit a fire under my clients' butts. Every day they'd ask, "Was that workout HAF?"

I highly recommend you develop an award for your clients. Ever since the HAF badge started my clients worked harder and canceled fewer workouts. They all wanted to win. The result? They all reached their goals faster. It also brought my clients together. I would catch them chatting in the gym, saying things like, "Have you been HAF this month?"

The HAF badge was also a physical object. I designed it (poorly) and would write the winner's name on it. He or she would usually display it on their fridge or mantle and show it off to their friends and family.

After all, who doesn't want to show off that they're HAF?*

9. Never be alone

Never let a client see you bored. In fact, don't let anyone see you bored. Nobody wants to work with a trainer who has too much time on his or her hands.

---

* When I started my website I created another award called the JARG, (Jon Award for Recognizing Greatness). I gave it to people who recognized that I was great.

Life's short. Be silly. Have fun.

Stay mobile. Stay engaged. Even if you genuinely have nothing to do, create the illusion that you're busy. If you're seen, be with people. If not, stay out of sight. If you look engaged and friendly and popular, people will be intrigued. Nobody wants to train with a bored trainer. Popularity begets popularity.

10. Build your own online community

Online communities are some of the most valuable social media assets you can own. All things change, of course, and one day this won't be true, but as long as everyone is still talking about Facebook or Instagram or the next disruptive thing, online groups can help your business.

A community's greatest value: Your reputation. Your group allows you to control the conversation, become the expert, lead by example, and prove you're an authority to a small yet very engaged group of people. Yes, there's a little bit of celebrity for you here, and that's part of the point.

A community's greatest risk: You run it poorly with mushy, ill-defined goals, substandard content, and no way to make members become advocates for you and your business.

Here are some quick tips on getting your online community up and running:

Come up with a winning name. A great group name

highlights who the group is for, makes people want to join, and encourages members to share the group within their own networks. A bad group name puts you on the defensive. For example, consider how many groups have names like "Lose Your Last 10 Pounds Challenge." While it communicates the purpose, these groups don't get shared because nobody shows off that they have 10 pounds to lose.

A good name identifies the audience (moms or dads, runners or lifters ...) and either communicates a benefit or elicits intrigue. The final word of the group name does the heaviest lifting: It needs to excite your target market by using language familiar to them and highlight the biggest benefit of group membership. At the time of writing, my two online communities hosted on Facebook are called Fit Pros Unite and Online Trainers Unite. Notice that they both end with the same word — the rally cry!

Start with three pieces of content.

About: In one or two lines, describe who the group is for and its goal.

Rules: "Always be kind, helpful, and respectful" is a good place to start, but the biggest one is probably "Spammers will be banned, no exceptions."

Group image: This should have the name of your group and your branding. It can include your company's logo, but it shouldn't be prominent. (You're the only one who cares about your logo.)

HOW "RUN WITH GINA" SERVES GINA MAURICIO'S ONLINE TRAINING BUSINESS

From Gina Mauricio, founder of
RunWithGina.com

I have a private Facebook group, Run with Gina, that complements my online training business and everything else I do as a fitness professional. Funny thing is, it didn't start that way.

I launched the group at the beginning of 2019 and put 25 clients in there. It was intended to be an accountability/support group so my clients could all see how the others were doing in their half- or full-marathon training. And it is that, but by happy accident it ended up being a lot more. Here's how:

— I welcomed unexpected guests. *When I started the group, I screwed up the settings and didn't list myself as the lone moderator, so my clients were able to add their own people, their running friends. I realized how awesome this was pretty quickly, because all of a sudden these friends have a front-row seat for how I interacted with my clients. Instant window shoppers. If someone missed a training session, for example,*

*she'd admit it to the group and the non-clients
would see how I worked with everyone to keep
them on track and encouraged. The result: A lot
of those window shoppers became clients.*

— I don't sweat the numbers. *A lot of people
think social media is a numbers game, the more
people engaged, the better. Not in this group.
I know I have 227 members, but that's only
because I looked it up for this occasion.*

*It's not a matter of quantity. It's all about having
good people who want to interact. You'll get three
kinds of people in a group like this: lurkers who
just scroll through and don't interact, engagers
who comment on everything, and the middle type
who just say something basic like, "Good job."
I prefer to have as many positive, enthusiastic
members as possible because they pull the lurkers
and introverts out of their shells to interact.
They fuel each other's fires. When someone sees
someone else succeeding, they wonder,* hey, how
can I make that happen? *And they join the
conversation.*

— I let the group be the group. *A good group
of quality members runs itself. It's not a time
suck for me. For example, all my runners are
on an app and training platform, so if someone
has a tech problem with that, someone else in the*

group probably has the answer for them. I get notifications on posts and comments, but I don't have to respond to every single one, and I don't. The members have gotten to know each other very well, so it's not time-consuming for me at all. That's the mark of a healthy group.

— Sometimes the group becomes a big testimonial page featuring me, and I let it. *I'm generally a modest person, but after I was featured in a* Runner's World *article for the work I've been doing, I received 70 messages in the private group.*

A few of those people ended up buying and one of them went on the page and told her story. Everyone started commenting like, "welcome to the group," "you're in the right place," "Gina's gonna take care of you." It was all about blowing smoke up my butt. I almost felt bad for the people in the group who didn't know me well. Is this place all Gina all the time? *Nope, not always. But I had to accept that 70 people just said something awesome about me. Each one a testimonial. So there's a bit of celebrity to running a group like this. Be prepared to be gracious about it because it's your group and you'll be the leader and expert.*

11. Informally invite people to join you in your own activities

*From Dustin Maher, founder of Dustin Maher Fitness and Fit Moms for Life (**dustinmaherfitness.com**)*

Some trainers are great at bringing people together. You can do this in a formal way with formally organized, formally announced events and do really well. You can do this with social media. It all works. The stuff I do, however, is a lot more informal. That feels natural to me, so there's nothing fake or staged about it.

Sometimes it's a simple invitation: *Hey, I'm going for a run at XYZ park on Sunday morning, who wants to join me?* Some of my clients will come out and bring friends. It's fun, no-stress, and prospects get to meet me and ask questions, or just hang. I'll also invite people to sign up for races.

My thing is sharing whatever journey I'm currently on. I signed up for an Ironman triathlon without knowing how to swim. Now I do open swims with whoever wants to come. I've done stair racing (running up skyscrapers) and fitness modeling. I tell my stories and always share what I learn, even if it's embarrassing. I'm honest and open about my fears. And I'm always happy to answer questions.

The sharing is key and it costs nothing. Everyone has their hang-ups and I put mine out there, which leads to so many conversations. And inviting people on a run? I'm going anyway, might as well go with a fun group. All of it, every share of time or funny stories or answering someone's questions, lets people see what I'll be like to work with. They see that it's truly a "join us and we'll support you" deal.

As trainers, we tend to put ourselves on pedestals. I'd rather be relatable. That's better for my brand.

12. Track your leads and don't let any fall through the cracks

From Jodi Rumack, cofounder of Accelerator Circle (***acceleratorcircle.com***)

If you're doing things right, you should amass an impressive number of prospects even if they don't all sign up for training. The ones who don't? Hey, they're still warm leads and you need to be a very friendly-but-determined bulldog about never letting them go.

The key? Develop a systematic process for tracking all your leads. And stick to it. That second part there is the most important. The best lead-tracking system in the world is pointless if you don't use it. I'll show you how the process works here, and offer some downloadable resources, as well ...

The thing about warm leads: They aren't just names and numbers and email addresses you collect. They're people you want to work with. So even if they haven't signed up, each follow-up with them is a chance to further develop your relationship. That's the approach that will earn you more goodwill and trust, as opposed to soulless follow-ups designed to extract money.

Let's go chronologically (see the flowchart at the end of this section for a complete breakdown) ...

A lead comes in. Could be via phone, email, or someone you meet. Add this person to your lead tracking form.[*] Fill out as many details as you can at the time, knowing you'll fill in more info as time goes by and you stay engaged.

Week 1	# of people I talked to (got their goals) today	# of consultations booked today	# consultations done today	# people who bought PT today	Booking %	Show %	Close %
Sunday	N/A	N/A	N/A	N/A	N/A	N/A	N/A
Monday	7	2	1	0	29%	50%	0%
Tuesday							
Wednesday							
Thursday							
Friday							
Saturday							
Total					29%	50%	0%

Week 2	# of people I talked to (got their goals) today	# of consultations booked today	# consultations done today	# people who bought PT today	Booking %	Show %	Close %
Sunday	N/A	N/A	N/A	N/A	N/A	N/A	N/A
Monday	7	4	2	0	57%	50%	0%
Tuesday							
Wednesday							
Thursday							
Friday							
Saturday							
Total					57%	50%	0%

Week 3	# of people I talked to (got their goals) today	# of consultations booked today	# consultations done today	# people who bought PT today	Booking %	Show %	Close %
Sunday	N/A	N/A	N/A	N/A	N/A	N/A	N/A
Monday	8	5	3	1	63%	60%	33%
Tuesday							
Wednesday							
Thursday							
Friday							
Saturday							
Total					63%	60%	33%

Call and email the prospect within 24 hours of first contact. Ideally, you want someone to come in for a consult within three days, but be an

---

*Every trainer should use lead tracking sheets and a monthly business tracker to manage leads. Don't have those? Try ours. Download our free tracking forms at **theptdc.com/leadtrackingform**.*

accommodating scheduler. If you get voicemail, leave a message and follow up in two or three days. Same with email.

Let prospects know how *excited* you are to work with them. Tone of voice is extremely important, particularly over the phone (this also applies to the confirmation call you make the night before the consult). You want to be sincere and fired up, but not over the top.

What if the prospect is a no-show for the consult/ free workout? Call the prospect 15 minutes after the session was supposed to start. If he answers, ask if everything is okay and whether he'd like to come in or reschedule. If you get voicemail, ask him to call you back between X and Y times. Tell him you'll also follow up via email. If you don't connect, follow up again in two weeks.

Update your lead tracking sheet and monthly business tracker. This step is easy to skip. Don't. Even leads that feel ice cold can one day convert out of nowhere.

Continue to follow up. Friendly check-ins are crucial to keeping leads warm. Follow the flowchart process and maintain your tracking forms. Again, this is the stuff that all successful trainers do, but no one wants to talk about because it just ain't sexy and offers no instant gratification. But it's key to a thriving business. Don't let up!

THE TAKEAWAY

Be willing to embrace the unsexy, underrated things you need to do to get clients and you'll have far more success than the trainers who don't want to be bothered. Do these things consistently over time the same way you'd encourage a client to stick to a workout plan. You'll love the results.

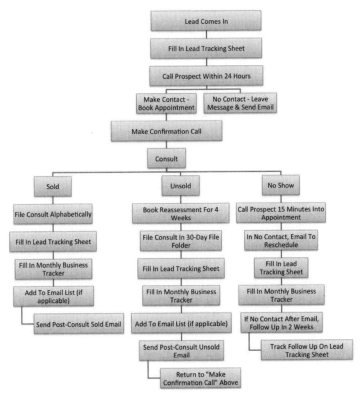

This flowchart illustrates the complete care-and-feeding of a lead. Let this become your process. And don't skimp on the details. Prospects who show interest may take months to finally sign on. Do you want to miss their business because you stopped following up? I'll say what people don't want to hear: Processes like these separate the successful trainers from the frustrated ones. Download a copy of this chart at
theptdc.com/leadflowchart.

CHAPTER 6

Fast One-Off Promotions for New Clients

"The purpose of a business is to create a customer."

—Peter Drucker

The most successful trainers always have something cool and exciting in the pipeline. This attracts new clients, of course, but also invigorates the day-to-day for you.

The good news? Every idea in this chapter works. The catch? You need to find out if they'll work for *you*.

That's the danger of having so many fantastic ideas. You want to do them all. I get it. That's been one of the great lessons I've had to learn both as a trainer and later as founder. My instinct has always been to try as much as possible, as soon as possible. That enthusiasm is awesome, it drives you, but I've learned the hard way that too much of a good thing ain't so good.

It's simple: Unfocused attention on too many bright ideas is much worse than focused attention on one basic idea. Like I said, all of these things you're about to read work, but I suggest you pick one that really fits you, focus on it, and crush it.

Yes, you can add new ideas later — repeat: the most successful trainers always have something new and exciting in the pipeline — but you need to focus like a laser, not a shotgun.

13. Build promos on the heels of holidays (even the weird ones)

I'm putting this one right here, leading off, because it ties in so tightly with a lot of what's to come in this chapter. Some of the most fruitful one-off promotions will spring from one essential source: the calendar.

Trainers underutilize the calendar, in my experience. Sure, you keep a schedule for clients, meetings, events, all of that. But I'm talking about using your calendar as a promotional weapon, as a 365-day source of potential one-off promotions.

Of course, holidays are the first line of offense. New year, new you. Pick your calendar-y reason to slim down: Valentine's Day, summer, wedding season, homecoming, the holidays.

But there's so much more you could tie into. Think of all the "days" on that calendar.

- How about doing some nice public display of affection for all your clients' birthdays?
- Do some "break the routine" event on Groundhog Day.
- Unleash your creativity for Friday the 13ths, April Fools', Mardi Gras, Cinco de Mayo, and Super Bowl Sunday.
- And what about all those manufactured events that become hashtags like National Cheeseburger Day, or Dog/Cat Day, or why not have a Take Your Kid to the Gym Day with sweat-inducing games and activities?

That's the calendar, folks. A deep well of ideas if you just put your brain on it.*

The obvious advice would be to sit down near the end of each year with next year's calendar in front of you and start filling it up with great one-offs. Plot the whole dang year ahead of time. And you should. But I also recommend going farther than that. Set aside time to check the calendar throughout the year, as well. You never know what new ideas might pop up, like a dog owner meet-and-greet for gym members and friends of members.

---

*Websites exist that break down the year's holidays, observances, and weird occasions. Try **HolidaysCalendar.com.**

14. Host community events and become the center of attention

Sponsoring a big, splashy local event is a great way to attract new prospects. The question is: What to do and how to do it successfully? Lots of potential here, and variables. As you brainstorm possibilities for your area, consider the following story ...

At the PTDC, we pay a lot of lip service to the idea of abundance. It makes a lot of sense in theory. Who would argue against the value of helping others succeed, even if they're your "competition?" I say it a lot: If you think you're competing in this business, you've already lost. It's at the core of what we teach.

I say that knowing it's easier said than done, especially if you're a trainer in a gym seeing other trainers land clients you know you'd work well with, or a gym owner watching other gyms in your area thrive while you hustle for every prospect.

That's why I was happy to get a Facebook message from Ben Boudro, owner of Xceleration Fitness in Auburn Hills, Michigan:

> *Hi Jon,*
>
> *Your* Fitness Marketing Monthly* *inspired me*

---

* *Just a reminder what FMM is: In* Fitness Marketing Monthly, *we brought together the brightest minds in the fitness industry and published more than 200,000 words of world-class, deep-dive marketing advice tailored to fit pros and their daily challenges. The entire set is available at* **theptdc.com/fmm.**

> *to do something crazy. One of the articles was*
> *how to host a local seminar. So I ran with it and*
> *came up with an event I'm hosting.*
>
> *We're inviting four gym owners in our area to*
> *come in and present their workouts and all they*
> *have to offer. Four different gyms who technically*
> *are our competitors.*
>
> *Why? Well, I thought it would be a novel idea,*
> *and also because I like the other gym owners and*
> *I'd like to help people out who need to find a gym,*
> *but aren't sure where to start.*

To which I replied:

> *Ben, this is fantastic, I love the concept.*
> *Whenever you bring people together and become*
> *that bridge, your own status increases. You're the*
> *obvious expert. This is basically how I built the*
> *PTDC, by the way.*

Showcasing community events like this can be a powerful recruitment tool, for all the reasons I just said, but also as a differentiator for you among local peers. There are some tricks* to this, however.

Ben's showcase was billed as the One-Hour Gym Speed-Dating Workout. Here's a snippet from the promo:

---

* The tricks for a traditional event are a little different than those for a charity fitness event, which we'll cover in a moment. There is some overlap, however, so you can learn from both models.

You Might Not Find Love...
But You Will Find A Gym You Can Fall In Love With!

Meet & Sweat with the best of the best
Fitness Pro's in Metro-Detroit!

What is this?

This will be a 1-hour workout where you can get a taste of 4 different coaches from 4 of the best gyms in Metro-Detroit.

You'll spend 15-minutes with each coach and then rotate!

Each rotation will allow you to experience a different style of fitness so that you can find the best fit for you in 2019!

*Have you ever wanted to box?

*Do you want to see what Pure Barre is all about?

*Have you ever trained with Body of Learning in Birmingham?

*Want to try out the #1 Boot Camp in Metro-Detroit?

You will do all of that in just 1-hour at this once in a lifetime event!

The simple digital promo flyer Ben used to spread word of his "speed dating" workout showcase event that brought together local fitness companies. A true example of why operating with abundance is a great strategy.

One of the key elements here: All the gyms offer something different. It's a great mix. No workout works for everybody. We all know that. But knowing it and acting on it the way Ben did is extremely rare. Inviting his potential customers to test-drive different approaches to fitness, including those of his competitors, is more than an example of abundance. It shows his passion for helping his neighbors by giving them a chance to pick the approach that's best for them. The pitch also earned him a four-minute segment on Fox 2 Detroit.

There's more to this story, however. Sign-ups were okay, but not gangbusters. So Ben had to pivot, and his pivot worked because he was paying attention:

> *Update for you! I got us on Fox 2 Detroit to*
> *promote it. We got about 23 sign-ups. But I*
> *realized people have been more enticed when*
> *I mentioned Lululemon would be there with*
> *clothing giveaways.*
>
> *I switched my marketing to focus on that and we*
> *got eight sign-ups in the next hour.*

Fortunately, one of the participating studio owners, Kristin Batchik, is a Lululemon ambassador who could hook them up with free samples. And everyone loves a giveaway, especially when it's Lululemon. Often when you do the right things, good stuff happens that you could never have predicted. See what happens when you operate with abundance?

The results: 52 people bought tickets, four area gyms co-ran the workout, seven vendors attended, and Ben sold seven memberships/upsells. They even had a photographer come out and shoot the event for free. Ben also built a relationship with the Fox News affiliate and is now the local expert featured regularly on the network.

The upshot: With zero advertising budget, Ben gained seven new members, added value to his network, got free high-quality photography for his studio, became a local media expert, and had fun.

That's how you bring a good event together.

15. **Run a charity fitness event**

*From Luka Hocevar, founder of Vigor Ground Fitness and Performance (**lukahocevar.com**)*

Throw an epic event, raise money for a good cause, and generate a ton of qualified leads at the same time. What's not to like? Running a great event isn't a quickie thing, however. You'll need at least several weeks of prep, then another week afterward to follow up with leads and get them through your doors, plus getting the money you raised out to the respective charities.

A charity event can cost you as much as you want. You'll have to invest time, of course, but volunteers and sponsorships can keep your business costs at zero. You can also pony up for extras like paid press release distribution, a DJ, and food out of pocket. How much or how little is up to you. Here's a basic step-by-step process for launching a charity event (for this example, a bootcamp):

Step 1. Commit to making it awesome. No one wants to run an "okay" or "good" event. You want your event to be EPIC — and that takes commitment to both the event and the charity you've chosen. The weekly charity bootcamps we host at my gym, Vigor, typically bring in between 40 to 80 people every Saturday (though we've thrown some bigger events). This method has been hands-down our most effective strategy for business growth. That said, running a successful event doesn't just happen. Be ready to work.

Step 2. Learn your legal responsibilities about earning money for your charity. I suggest going local before going national. It makes a bigger difference in your community and bonds people together, while also encouraging support from local businesses. Think about how you'll collect money for the charity safely and legally. A few considerations:

- We collect everything by check and cash, and we have a Square reader for cards — however, we strongly encourage cash and check so we don't lose donations to processing fees. We've also set up payment links for people when they wanted to donate but couldn't come to the bootcamp.

- Understand the legal implications of fundraising. I recommend you check with your accountant because different states have different rules when it comes to promoting charity events and how you phrase them. For example, we had to switch from "charity bootcamp" to "bootcamps for a cause" due to legal issues around the wording.

- Decide how much you will give away and be prepared to be crystal clear about it. We give away everything raised, 100 percent gross. I cover my expenses out of pocket. While how much you give away is up to you, I prefer to say that every penny raised is contributed — and deliver on that promise.

Step 3. Establish the basics. Name, timing, and the size you're aiming for. Set a participant goal number for yourself that's realistic yet suitable for the size of your venue. And don't be afraid to start small. Our first only had seven people. That was a deliberate choice to get the kinks out before growing the program.

Step 4. Design the event. The easiest way to discover what you really want to do is to simply ask, "Why?" Write out exactly why you're doing this, who you're doing it for, and the specific outcomes you hope to achieve.

Anytime I related my feelings and emotions about why this is so important to me, the event was so much more successful. This understanding will also help define your marketing efforts. The exercise program should be the easiest part to create, assuming you're used to designing bootcamps or group training classes. Think of ways to make the event special, challenging, or creative. Some ideas:

- Bring in a DJ, "hype person," local celeb, or comedian to emcee and help kick things off. Better still, a local celeb to work out with the group.

- Vendors and sponsors can add freebies and fun to your event with no extra cost to you. Local businesses love exposure. Popular eateries or watering holes can provide food and drink for an afterparty.

- Hire a photographer/videographer. Document for posterity (and social).

- Alert local media for possible coverage.

- The key: Be creative about generating hype.

Step 5. Never let your sales pitch overshadow the event. My rule: No selling during a charity event. You want to generate business from the event, for sure. Just be classy about how you do it.

We have people fill out a waiver form when they show up that includes name, email, physical address, and phone. After the event, we politely follow up with a "thank you" for helping the cause, and offer them a trial week of our programs. Many people ask to sign up simply because they love the program. Others keep coming every Saturday and end up joining a little bit later when they realize they need more than just the weekly bootcamp to get results. Either way, we get a ton of leads, and above all, we get to help the causes we care about.

16. Gather emails with "of the day" promos

An ongoing "of the day" promotion is an easy way to get people to sign up for your content, and hopefully your training. When you meet a new prospect, as you wrap up the conversation, offer them an opportunity for a free recipe or exercise of the day. In exchange for an email address, you'll send recipes, exercises, or other healthy tips. The key: Your content has to provide value and expect nothing in return. Great daily content keeps you top of mind and this list will prove key to growing your business through ongoing nurturing and converting.

17. Create a transformation contest or challenge[*]

From Ryan Ketchum, business coach and marketing expert

Transformation contests are big money and a big way to draw attention to your brand in the fitness world. I built my previous business, Force Fitness and Performance, to more than 400 clients using transformation contests as the main lead generator. It's very easy to screw up, however. I know because I've made many mistakes myself. I'll show you how to avoid them.

In my previous business, we'd run six to eight transformation contests a year. One time we ran an eight-week transformation contest that got us 125 new clients signed up by the end of it. The registrations alone brought in more than $20,000. So, yeah, you can really drive new business this way. (It's also a great way to show people that you're really good at getting them the results they want.)

Here are some key ingredients for a successful transformation contest:

---

[*] *Understand the difference: A contest offers competition with a prize at the end. Challenges are simply undertaken by individuals or groups for, well, the challenge of it. Some trainers like to run contests that crown clear winners, others prefer a straight challenge. Both get proven results and client engagement, so it all comes down to the trainer's personal preference.*

—Create your "hook" and deadline. One of the biggest reasons transformation contests work so well is the deadline. You need two: a deadline to register and a deadline to hit the weight-loss or fitness goal.

Take a quick look at the calendar for a holiday or event (like the start of summer) that's at least several weeks away. This date needs to be six to eight weeks out for a shorter contest, or 12 to 16 weeks for a longer one.

When I used to plan out my yearly marketing calendar at Force Fitness, I'd set up two longer transformation contests each year and fill in the rest with shorter-term transformation challenges or contests. The two big contests were after the New Year, usually starting around the first week of February; and in the fall, around the start of the school year. These proved to be the best times to get people motivated without interruption from other holidays.

Give yourself three to four weeks to market your program. Once you have the end date (which also helps you figure out your "hook," or the main draw), you can work backward to determine the start date and marketing calendar.

The next step is determining your hook, or the theme of your transformation contest. This is an important step that I've messed up more than once, so don't take it lightly.

Your hook will attract people and let them know this transformation contest is for them. Typically you want to hit on emotion, which will dictate your marketing

TRANSFORMATION CONTEST HOOKS

SUMMER SLIMDOWN	**AMAZING ABS**
HOLIDAY SURVIVAL	**LEAN BODY**
NEW YEAR, NEW YOU	**FIT 2B STRONG**
MEMORIAL DAY MELTDOWN	**LIVING LEAN**
SPRINT TO SPRING BREAK	**RAPID FAT LOSS**
ROCK YOUR JEANS	**EASY ABS**
HOT BODY EXPRESS	**BLAST THE FAT**
TONE EVERY ZONE	**TIGHTER TUSH**
DROP A DRESS SIZE	**PHOTOFIT**
LITTLE BLACK DRESS	**FIT NOT FAT**

Samples of potential themes and hooks for your transformation contest. Feel free to use any of these or adapt however you like.

message, right down to the promotional emails and sales copy. Think of the hook as a reason for people to sign up for the contests.

Now that you have your hook and the timeline for your contest, you need to determine if you will offer prizes or if this will be a straightforward challenge. You also need to figure out the programming offered and how you'll take registrations.

—**Don't complicate your registrations.** Generally, you want an online sales page and online marketing. However, don't think if you can't set up a sales page you can't run a big contest. I ran my first ever 100-person contest without a sales page and took all registrations via phone or email. It was a lot more work, but it can be done.

For maximum efficiency, build a sales page that links to your payment processing system. At Force Fitness, we'd link our sales page to our Mindbody system to take payments immediately. This is hands-down the best way to take registrations, but it isn't the only way. It's just very effective because you can get people to commit immediately.

If you can't collect money online (Paypal makes this easy), simply ask for a name and email and perform a manual follow-up to collect payment. Don't make this too complicated. Here's a sample name and email registration page I created at Force Fitness. Once customers entered the info, it directed them to a purchase page using Mindbody.

If You Are Ready To Drop Fat Fast and Feel Better Than Ever Before Register For Your 7-Day Rapid Fat Loss Detox for just $29 NOW!

Enter Your Name...

Enter Your Email...

Register Now!

—Keep your program offerings simple. In my experience, too many options for joining your transformation contest can lead to poor numbers. Ask yourself: *What program would I put someone on to get him the best results?* That's the program you start with.

I always had three offerings covering a range of price points. Any more than that would get too confusing and tough to manage. The first offering was our lowest price for basic members, usually something like group personal training for two to three days per week. The second offering was a midrange offer for personal training two to three days per week. A combo offering of personal and group training was our highest-priced offering for four to five days per week.[*]

I suggest placing the one you want most people to do in the middle of the range. Marketing psychology suggests the middle pricing makes that option the most appealing. (There's also no harm in offering only two options.)

—Use price to guide who signs up. You can take two approaches when pricing your transformation contests: low cost/high volume or high cost/lower volume. Mixing them up throughout the year is a great strategy and one that I have had a lot of success with in the past. Keeping the longer six- or eight-week transformation

---

[*] *A great way to add additional value (and revenue) is to offer a nutrition component as a relevant upsell to participants in the challenge. This could be part of a bigger package or an add-on. Either way, it's pure profit.*

contests at a high price and the 21- or 28-day challenges at a lower price helped me balance things out.

—**Determine your prizes.** The most obvious (and best) prize is cold, hard cash. Let's first address the fact that people are getting amazing results, or at least they should be, which is the ultimate prize (which is why challenges work just as well as contests).

Examples of prizes include:

- Cash $$$$$
- Getaways
- Joint venture offerings
- Other prizes (physical objects)

If you're good with numbers, you can easily figure out how much cash to offer. Take your average registration fee and multiply it by the number of contestants you think you'll get. For instance, if your average registration fee is $149 and you want 35 people, you're left with $5,215 ($149 × 35). In this case, I would easily be comfortable with giving away $2,500 as prize money, considering the primary goal of the challenge is lead generating. That still leaves me with $2,500-plus to pay for staff and marketing expenses, as well as the bonus of any new client conversions that come out of the contest.

If a new client is worth $199 per month to you and they stick around for 12 months, that's $2,388 per new client to your business. If you convert, say, 30 percent of those 35 sign-ups to new clients, that's 10 to 11 new clients worth at least $23,880 to your business in the next year. I would pay $2,500 to get $23,880 in return every day of the week!

—Get the word out. A lot of contest marketing is sales copy, networking, and paid ads, but let me just tell you that you should play to your strengths. If you're good with people and have a strong network, for example, leverage it. If you are good with Facebook ads and email marketing, leverage it. It's okay to try new things, and if needed, get someone to set them up for you.

I would start with the following:

- Your current clients
- Your email list of non-clients
- Your clients for referrals
- Your business connections and joint ventures
- Press releases and media contacts
- Paid ads through Google, Facebook, or anywhere else you've had success

No matter your marketing plan, make sure to make the most of it. Once you start getting results with your transformation programs, marketing them becomes much easier on social media, as the results tend to go viral and word gets out about your awesome event. Add an extra promo punch by developing rewards the winners can show off, like one of those giant checks, for example. Have the winner pose for a pic. Then you can use that in promotions the next time.

WHAT I LEARNED FROM A LITTLE BLACK DRESS (LBD)

From Alicia Streger, founder of Fit Pro Essentials (**FitProEssentials.com**)

The Little Black Dress Project started as a passion project. I wanted to go deeper, create more connection with my clients, and really empower them to live their best lives. It was a huge success, and quickly became my signature program. I sold my fitness business after nine years in 2016, and now I work strictly business to business (B2B), offering The LBD Project 1.0 and 2.0 to other fitness pros. Now more than a thousand coaches all over the world run The Little Black Dress Project. Here's how it all happened:

—It sprang from an intimate understanding of my clients. *At the time, about 80 percent of my clients were women. I noticed this underlying belief that many of them didn't feel worthy of taking time for themselves or putting themselves first. They were so busy doing everything for everyone else, that their own goals and health suffered. They didn't just need more tools in their tool belt. They wanted connection and to be a part of something special, and have a plan to achieve their goals. So I wanted to create a program that not only gave them the tools and resources they needed to succeed, but give them an opportunity to connect with other women, have FUN, and celebrate them for the amazing women they already are!*

—It had a sexy hook. *Challenges are EVERYWHERE right now. You need a specialized "hook" targeted to a specific audience. A general challenge won't set you apart anymore. The LBD Project isn't even called a challenge. It's The Little Black Dress Project and it helps transform lives. Women are attracted to it because not only do they want to feel confident and rock a little black dress, they want to be a part of something special and unique.*

—The more we encouraged people to bring in friends, the better it worked. *People who signed up with friends or family almost always got better results, for obvious reasons. But that became a true incentive when we talked to new prospects. Whenever anyone signed up, we'd ask, "Do you have a friend or family member who has similar goals that may want to join the program with you?" We'd talk about success rates being higher with that kind of support and even offer an incentive if they brought other people in.*

—ALWAYS wow and overdeliver. *This will truly make you stand out and create raving fans. Clients expect the usual: workouts, check-ins, and the like. They also expect you to be your awesome self. But the more little surprises you can bring, the more unexpected celebrations or love notes or quick-hit moments that bring smiles, the more memorable your program becomes. It's all about the details.*

—When your challenge gains traction, be ready to offer more. *The LBD Project (the original) is a fine-tuned program. We ran it so many times that we knew exactly what worked and what didn't over the years. I launched 2.0 simply because people wanted more — more workouts, new recipes, fresh content. The whole thing is new. But it follows the same structure. People just wanted to keep going and so I had to have something ready for them. Always anticipate your clients' needs. The goal is to be so in tune with your clients that you know what they need, before they even know that they need it.*

—Throw a great party at the end. *The Little Black Dress parties became a major selling point for the program. The event gives people something to work toward, aside from measurements, feeling amazing, and reaching some of their goals. Everyone gets a chance to wear their little black dresses, we give awards, and everyone celebrates the previous six weeks. We also let people bring guests to the party so friends, family, and spouses could support and join in on the fun. That led to even more people signing up. It was an amazing client-getting strategy. And you know what? I'm certain some people joined just for the party at the end. And that's just fine.*

18. Leverage local public speaking to get lots of clients in one fell swoop

From Igor Klibanov, founder of Fitness Solutions Plus (**fitnesssolutionsplus.ca**)

I started my training business in 2011 out of school with a degree in kinesiology, which meant I knew nothing about marketing and sales. I was an entrepreneur, I had my own training business, but I thought being a good trainer would be enough to get me referrals.

Reality check: I was *really* wrong. I read a ton of marketing and business books, and trust me, small business marketing is very different from big business marketing. And every small business marketing book I read said "public speaking, public speaking, public speaking." So I gave it a shot.

My first 40 public speaking gigs got me no clients whatsoever. That sounds bad, but people were signing up for my newsletter, so I thought people might buy in over months or even years. Still, I needed clients *now*. I had all these potential clients just sitting there at my talks. There had to be a better way.

Then I made one simple adjustment and *everything* changed: After every talk, I'd been offering people a gift certificate for a discounted session that expired in two weeks. At my next talk, I changed the expiration date from two weeks to 20 minutes after I finished speaking. The offer's off the table when I leave the building.

The first time I tried it, nearly 40 percent of the crowd signed up for a discounted initial assessment. *Urgency and scarcity changed everything.*

Now I do 45 to 50 speaking gigs per year, mostly at corporations, which keeps pace with how many qualified staff I can hire to handle all the leads. If I did more, I wouldn't be able to keep up with demand. Right now I have 14 qualified trainers working for me. I could hire lower-quality staff and do more gigs, but I don't want to risk my reputation in any way.

My approach to speaking has evolved over the years, but here are the main things I've learned ...

—Information and education fail. My goal starting out was to educate and inform. And people tuned out. I believe they were either overwhelmed with info or they thought, *Okay, I know enough to try this out myself.* Either way, I was being excluded from the transaction. Now my purpose is selling and my results reflect that. Education is a side effect. Related point: I used to hate talking about myself, but I added an introduction to my talks and my sales improved. So that's a key component.

—Seed liberally. I try to include things that make the audience wonder, *How can I work with him?* without my specifically saying, "Here's how you can work with me." I seed with lots of case studies: "Here's my client Jennifer, she lost 45 pounds." That's seeding, preparing the audience for a pitch.

—Understand what generates *your* profit. Some speakers charge a fee and make a nice revenue stream out of it. That's fine. I'm happy to forego a $1,000 or even $2,000 speaking fee to have the opportunity to sell more than $2,000 worth of personal training. Sure, I'm taking the chance that no one signs up, but most of the time it works out in my favor.

—Warm 'em up, part one. Before I do a gig at a corporation, everyone attending gets a PDF of my book ahead of time so they know who I am. That makes a cold audience a warm audience. The catch: The earlier I can send it the better. If I have a speaking engagement booked in two months, I'll send the PDF and my subsequent newsletters two months out.

—Warm 'em up, part two. I arrive 15 to 30 minutes early and engage with some people before I start. I ask what they want out of the talk. I get *them* talking. I ask them for questions beforehand and then run through some during the event. The key is to engage before you take the stage. Then I have them sign up for my email list during the talk.

—Bring guests. I always invite a few people to come with me to the talk, mostly other HR people from companies I'm trying to land or prospects I'm trying to convert.

—Target the right audience with the right offer at the right time. My ideal client is female, single (divorced or never married), lives in the greater Toronto area, and is 20 or more pounds overweight. I tailor my pitches to attract that audience and when the gig starts I use language friendly to that audience.

—Location matters. A talk 15 kilometers from your gym won't go as well as a talk 5 kilometers from your gym. Proximity = convenience and it's huge. My company offers remote training and we serve a large area, so it's less of a determinant for me.

—Cold emailing is better than cold calling. You'll have to go in cold to get a gig at some point. A call inevitably means being cycled through a phone system that always ends in voicemail. That sucks up a lot of time and voicemails are easy to ignore. Emails take seconds to send. For corporate pitches, I include the HR manager, the CEO, and COO. That way even if the HR person disregards my email, upper management might not and will tell HR to reach out to me.

Here's an example of a real pitch email that got me booked:

> *Hello,*
>
> *I am writing in hopes of finding the appropriate person who handles lunch and learns.*
>
> *I also wrote to [PERSON 1] and [PERSON 2] in that pursuit. If it makes sense to talk, let me know how your calendar looks for a quick, 5-10 minute phone call.*
>
> *Fitness Solutions Plus helps companies boost morale and employee engagement by providing lunch and learns on fitness, nutrition, hormones, and healthy aging. We tailor our talks to our audience to make sure that there is something directly relevant, interesting, and immediately applicable. Companies often see an improvement in productivity, energy levels, and mental clarity. In the past, I've provided lunch and learns for RBC, IBM, Intact Insurance, and others.*
>
> *If you are the appropriate person to speak with, what does your calendar look like, for a quick,*

five to 10 minute phone call? If not, who do you
recommend I talk to?

Thanks,

Igor Klibanov

**—Your first few gigs should be confidence
builders.** I did my first few speaking gigs at local high
schools. Expect nothing from them. If you bomb, it's no
big deal.

—Track every talk. I use an Excel document that
includes the name of the company, how many attended,
age range, demographics, how many converted into a
discounted session, and how many of those converted
into paying clients. That way I can see which talks are
profitable and which are unprofitable, and that shows
me tweaks I can make to improve results.

Date	Company/Occasion	Topic	Approx. Audience Size	Location	Audience Demographic

—Have a few different talks to offer. I always
include different talks in my pitch emails, which has
improved my book rate. I compete with myself by
testing new talks to see if they can beat the results of
my old talks.

19. Offer a ping-pong ball challenge

Put a jar full of ping-pong balls (or golf balls, or whatever works for you) out on a counter of a noncompeting, high-traffic business in your community.

In exchange for name and contact information, people can guess how many ping-pong balls are in the jar. The winner gets four weeks of free training (or whatever amount you feel works). But don't stop there. Every person who enters is a runner-up and gets one free session. You get a ton of leads. Not a bad deal for anyone.

20. Free upon completion scholarships

I've seen trainers offer scholarships a number of different ways. The most common is to make it free, but free isn't always best. In fact, it's a good example of something that sounds like it *should* be more effective than it actually is. Why? A free program can bring in the wrong kind of client and establish a bad precedent. Charging even just $1 will change the mentality of both client and trainer. People simply don't commit to training when it's cheap or free.

My favorite scholarship method is "free upon completion." It solves every problem in the scholarship model. It may result in a lower number of people, but you'll get much better results.

I first learned about "free upon completion" from U.K. online trainer Phil Harrison. Phil used this model with his online group transformation contests, but it works perfectly for scholarships, too. Here's how it works:

First, establish an attainable goal for your clients within a relatively short period of time. I recommend 30 days to a maximum of 45. Then tell clients the scholarship is free but there's a catch: It's only free if they do the work, because you only want to work with people ready to make a change. This sets the tone.

Price the scholarship at the same value as your coaching. For example, if you plan to charge $200 per month of coaching, then charge $200 for the scholarship. Explain to your clients that upon completion of the scholarship period, you'll return their $200 in full.

Technically, it's still free but taking the money up front has a few benefits:

- Clients who are ready to do the work — and likely to succeed in your program — naturally self-select.

- Money changes hands. You set a precedent in which the client pays you for your service. This makes it easier, psychologically, for them to pay for your services going forward after the scholarship is over.

- You maintain your value proposition. If you value your training at $200, then charging less, even in a scholarship, could hurt your chances of selling at that price point in the future.

- Converting scholarship participants into paying clients becomes easier at the end of 30 or 45 days. You know they're willing to pay for your services and now there's a precedent of doing so. What's more, you've drastically reduced their loss aversion, so they're easier to convert.

Let's spend a minute more on that last point. People tend to undervalue potential gain and overvalue potential loss. The gain is getting in better shape, looking great, having a longer life, increasing confidence, and whatever other benefits your training provides. The loss in this case is the money spent on achieving these things.

Rationally, the decision to get in shape should be an easy decision. Obviously health is worth all the money in the world. Say that to people and nine out of 10 will agree, but their actions may dictate otherwise. With the "free upon completion" method of charging for a scholarship you can make an attractive offer to your client a week or two before he finishes his 30 or 45 days: He gets his money back and can move on, or he can apply the money to his first month of coaching.

Technically the program is still free but after the money changes hands it feels like the cash is gone. As a result, the loss aversion is dampened. That money has already been out of the client's pocket for so long that he likely no longer misses it. That means he's more likely to put it toward an ongoing program with you. (Why ask for it back if it's already been "spent"?) Your conversion rates — as you take the person from "free" scholarship student to paying client — now skyrocket. Isn't psychology fun?

21. Launch a case study program

So simple it's genius: You let the world know you've developed a brand-new total-body transformation program and invite people to become part of a "select group" of case studies at a discounted rate.

This method can be effective because it taps into people's innate desire to be part of something special that isn't open to the general public. And at a discount, no less. After, say, four weeks or however long your case study lasts, participants will know you and have gotten results and will most likely continue on with you. Even if some don't, they'll remain warm leads you can stay in touch with.

22. Write a book and self-publish

This subject could take up a book all by itself because there are so many variables.* The bottom line: Being the "author of" something gives you instant credibility to laypeople and pros in the field. You can use it as a revenue stream, or a giveaway (downloadable PDFs are quick and easy), or leverage it to get speaking gigs,

---

* I have a free two-hour call on writing and publishing for fitness pros if you want to go deeper. Check it out:
theptdc.com/fitness-book-publishing.

interviews, and other media coverage.

The caveat: Your book has to be really, really, really good.

23. Build a marketing funnel

Marketing funnels sound so innovative and amazing when experts talk about them. Gets everyone excited. And funnels *can* work great — if you build one appropriate for your situation. The problem: Everyone's situation is different.

That's the challenge and pitfall of a funnel. *The nuances.*

Take email marketing software. Whichever suite you choose,* pick your poison, you need to understand the programs inside and out. For example, here's an unexpected piece you may not be aware of: What does a "day" mean to the system and what time zone is it set to? If your messaging system isn't in sync with that "day" definition, your customers will have a lousy experience.

That's the true danger: Even if you get clients into your funnel, one screwup could send dozens if not hundreds of people the wrong message. Next thing you know,

---

* I wish I could tell you what software to pick, but it's difficult to recommend a single product for funnels because there are so many options depending on what you need. Plus the software landscape changes so rapidly. What worked last year may be replaced this year. Your best bet is to investigate what trainers in similar situations have used and praised. Truth is, it's pretty hard to go wrong.

your customer support system is overloaded. Then you have to repair it all the way back to the initial glitch. Needle, meet haystack.

Another challenge: You have to know *all* your numbers. You have to trust those numbers. That's difficult when you're patching together different software packages. And that can get very expensive. High-end data tracking add-ons can quadruple software costs.

How about *this* trip to crazy town: We built a funnel for the Online Trainer Academy that has 10 automations and 122 steps (there are 17 automations, in fact, but we're not currently using seven of them). It's right for our situation. It gets results. We know our numbers down to the click and down to the penny and even then *it's really hard to make it work.*

Funnel software marketers leave out a lot of details, let me tell you.

Ya gotta start simple. A coach looking to level up to $5,000 to $10,000 per month just needs a basic lead generation system that collects contact info, automates booking, and takes payments. That's it.

The goal here: Automate the places a human doesn't need to be and maximize your presence in the places where a human *should* be. You want to eventually get a lead on the phone, because the phone is the best way to sell (aside from in-person, but that's an extra step).

One way a funnel can flow:

- A one-off promotion or some other incentive (free workout) entices a lead to enter her contact info into your system. Usually you're giving something of value in exchange for this info.

- Invite the lead to book a phone call with you.

- Your booking system should be automated so there's never any back-and-forth about "what date's good for you?" The lead sees all open slots and picks. Reminders happen automatically later.

- Throughout this process, give the lead every opportunity to book a phone call with you. Add nurture content to keep leads engaged who haven't booked. Let leads know what solution they need, but *not* that you are that solution.

- The call happens. A human shows up only when a human should, answering questions, assuaging fears.

This is just one way. So many possible iterations.

One thing you need to get right: Know how many phone calls you convert to clients. It's all part of one big cash equation:

How much you spend to acquire a lead --->
Number of phone calls you score from the lead pool --->
Number of phone calls you convert to clients.

If you know you need to boost your client roster by X new clients to cover costs and/or level up in income, and you know you usually convert five out of 10 phone leads, you now know how many leads you need to pull into your funnel to get X number of new clients and about how much it will cost.

Now all you need to do is entice those leads into your funnel through promotions, incentives, referrals, and the like.

In a way, funnels aren't brain surgery (though our OTA funnel may just qualify), but they do require time, money, and effort to do well. That's why simplicity is the key starting out. Later on? Your funnels can become more sophisticated, but only if your business *needs* sophistication.

10 WAYS TO INSTANTLY SET YOURSELF APART FROM OTHER TRAINERS

From Andrew Coates, founder of Andrew Coates Fitness
(**AndrewCoatesFitness.com**)

Shameless self-promotion can be the kiss of death in a service-oriented industry like fitness. The "ick" factor is sky-high. But there are ways you can promote yourself with class and authenticity. These ways will set you apart from other fit pros because, let me tell you, not many are doing them.

You'll employ one of the most obvious yet

underrated tools for getting new clients: the gym floor itself. That's where I'm coming from here, but understand that these ideas can easily be co-opted by online trainers in every digital and in-person interaction. The goal is the same for both: Establishing yourself as the stand-out professional in your facility and showcasing a consistent presence that causes people to approach and ask for your services.

Think of these as perpetual one-off promotions of your skills, bench-side manner, professionalism, and approachability.

24. Passive never sells

Everyone on a gym floor can see you whether or not you behave actively or passively, and over time people will process their impression of you based on that. What are they looking at?

- Your professional presence. *The basics like a neat and professional uniform (not removing parts of it when managers aren't around). Being clean and well groomed. Commonsense stuff that way too many coaches neglect for reasons that remain a mystery to me.*

- Standing and kneeling while coaching. *Or*

more specifically, not sitting down with lazy posture. Just as I was writing this, a client sent me the following: "Today I watched an inexperienced trainer 'teach' a client new to the gym ... terrible form, trainer sitting on his a**, not tracking anything ... I wanted to school him so bad!" Folks, if people judge you as a lazy trainer, they automatically rule you out as an option.

25. Look — and act — the part

Being in shape as a trainer is a controversial topic. People need to be who they are. But it's wise not to discount how judgmental humans are when they form snap first impressions. I know amazing trainers who aren't "ripped" or "jacked" and are always busy. So I like to put it this way: If you're a trainer who's not as in shape as our industry expects and you're struggling to be busy, make every effort to improve how visibly in shape you are on an ongoing basis.

We can be judged unfairly, and some may feel trainers lose credibility asking others to exercise and improve their nutrition when we ourselves aren't able to. An important note: Many trainers are inspired to work with others because of a personal transformation. Even if you are partway through a journey, sharing your story on your social media really helps people see how far you've come and makes you relatable to others with the same goal.

26. Never use a phone on the gym floor

Especially not with clients, as both your client and outside observers will think you're texting a hot date, even if you're using it to record client info.

I've used a tablet for years and it looks professional. I record client workouts, sessions, and schedules, and can film video easily. My clients love having their workouts emailed to them after.

A clipboard serves the same professional purpose. Remember, you will eventually have people approach you during a client session and ask about training with you. Make it easy for them to give you their contact info, either in the tablet or on paper. No one wants to see you working a phone in front of someone.

27. Lose yourself in engagement

Watch your client's movement intently. Study movement. I've learned more about coaching movement from studying every rep than from any textbook I've read. Mastery of your craft *comes from deliberate practice.*

Onlookers, who may themselves someday ask to train with you or send you referrals, can see your engagement. You can never predict when. I've had people approach me after watching for a few days or weeks, and some ask after years.

Most of all, clients quietly note your engagement with them. If you're fully engaged, they appreciate it and are far more likely to stick around. The best referral is a retained client.

28. No flirting

Just don't.

29. Smile at people

It's simple and powerful and not enough people do it. Wear a smile on the gym floor. Make eye contact. Be pleasant and make everyone's day a little better. People will remember how you made them feel.

I've worked alongside trainers who carry themselves with the stereotypical "resting b**** face." Know what? Members would talk among themselves about how unpleasant these staffers appeared. In my experience, those trainers only engaged people they believed would immediately *benefit them, and everyone noticed.*

30. No politics

Avoid politics and contentious social ideological topics in person and online, especially on your social media, no matter how safe you may feel on the moral high ground. You immediately risk offending upwards of half your potential client base. Plus, those discussions are time sucks that distract you from productive work. Not to mention the stress.

It doesn't matter how passionate you are about it, either. You risk branding yourself an activist instead of a fitness professional. Activism doesn't pay the bills. The overwhelming majority of the successful pros in our industry never touch such topics, and that should be enough to convince you.

This stuff always distracts and detracts from your mission to help as many people as possible. People from all parts of such ideological spectrums need help.

31. Leave judgmental attitudes behind

Okay, you're a fitness pro. What's your immediate reaction when you see an obese person eating junk food in public or someone smoking a cigarette outside a gym?

Be honest. You probably have a certain opinion of those people, whether you say it out loud or not. It's best you stop judging people, permanently.

Think about it this way: You have no idea where those two people are on a journey. The obese person may have just hit the 50-pounds-down mark that week and is enjoying a well-earned treat. The smoker may have cut down a lot and recently started to work out with every intention of quitting for good. Maybe there's more: Maybe the smoker is a recovering addict who's nine months sober.

Judgmental attitudes can kill your reputation. That also goes for posting "gym fail" videos or secretly filming people in a gym setting (even if you don't do it, watching them means you condone it).

Nothing will send away a potential new client faster than seeing you shame someone who doesn't know what they're doing.

32. Beware your superficial tendencies

Treat everyone as if they may someday become customers or referral sources, regardless of age, race, or any other superficial factor. One of the most enriching aspects of training a variety of people is learning about different cultures and places.

I've worked with clients from Denmark, Israel, Lebanon, India, Sri Lanka, Argentina, China, Mali, Honduras, Nicaragua, Brazil, plus every part of Canada. Especially important to note: People from some cultures are less easily sold if you don't first establish a relationship with them, but they're amazing at generating referrals for you once they've found a caring professional to believe in.

33. For students and newbie trainers: Target the right people

I've had a few practicum students and interacted with others (practicum means they're getting practical, first-hand experience at some point during their studies). Their practicum usually requires an assigned number of coaching hours with free clients, so these students hit up their young friends and coach the bare minimum required hours.

This is a huge blown opportunity.

Coaching isn't just a minimum requirement to check off. It's a chance to get in front of potential *clients and do a great job. Free clients may then become paying clients. The more touchpoints with free clients you make, the more chances one stays on after the student time is done.*

The best target for such free coaching isn't a trainer's young friends (who don't usually have the financial resources to pay for training) but their parents. *Invest in the relationship and you stand a much greater chance of retaining them past the mandatory free period. This principle works for generating regular clients, too.*

THE TAKEAWAY

One-off promotions are easy ways to generate buzz and excitement around your practice. Just make sure you give each one the proper focus. Too many promos at once and you risk lousy execution.

.

CHAPTER 7

Multimillion-Dollar Guerrilla Marketing Secrets Revealed!

by Mike Doehla, founder of Stronger U online nutrition coaching (strongeru.com)

"Do a good job and make sure everyone knows about it."

—Jonathan Goodman

Stronger U is a multimillion-dollar business with over 70 coaches built with virtually no paid advertising. More than 90 percent of our members come from word of mouth or guerrilla marketing.

That doesn't make me special, and certainly not visionary. I've simply been willing to try just about anything to bring positive attention to my business.

Everyone needs help with nutrition. That doesn't mean everyone is open to talking about it. I do everything I can to get people to "see" my brand and come to us for help with weight loss and intelligent eating. How do I do that?

That's a tough and easy question. Easy because, yeah, I relentlessly market. Tough because I've marketed my business in hundreds of ways, many of which I've forgotten.

That's guerrilla marketing. It's fluid. It's constant. It changes almost daily. Sometimes you're face-to-face with your audience. Sometimes you're a ghost leaving subtle and not-so-subtle hints.

The basics of it go back to what Jonathan Goodman says, "Do a good job and make sure everyone knows about it." Some fit pros have a big problem with that second part.

No one knows you're out there if you're scared to talk to people. Scared to promote your thing. Oh, I don't mean you're scared to advertise or be on social media or talk yourself up. I do mean you might not want to try all the goofy things I've tried and succeeded at.

There's a ton of failure and rejection in guerrilla marketing. You'll have little to no data on what works and what doesn't. Much of it's just, "Hey, let's try this."

It also saves your formal marketing from being stiff,

or staged, or fake. Guerrilla marketing comes straight from your gut, your soul, and your sense of fun (and sometimes absurdity).

Guerrilla marketing is a way to market without being obnoxious about it.

A good guerrilla marketing idea is a conversation starter, but a conversation *you* don't have to start. Almost like having someone doing the marketing for you. I create the idea — things just pop into my head — and I'm like, *How can I get someone to think about us in this situation?*

You're not cold calling. Don't think of these strategies as hard, complex, or inconvenient. For me, this is the fun stuff. You're doing unusual things that encourage people to know you and find you without even being present (sometimes). The introvert's dream, really.

I have a few rules for healthy guerrilla marketing. They're really simple (and hopefully you've adopted some form of them already) ...

—A *willingness to try anything.* Make a game of it. Embrace your creative, playful side.

Yes, creativity requires vulnerability. You're putting yourself out there. People don't want to do that ... but try it. I grew up as a super-shy kid. Embracing this mindset brought me out of my shell. I'll have conversations with random people now. When I was younger that would make me almost pass out. Now I just throw it out there. Some people won't like me, but there are people out there who need help and if I'm quiet they won't get it.

—A *drive to be genuine*. One rule at Stronger U: We never contribute to the BS in this industry.

We're in the business of selling people a better life. We're not trying to trick anyone. Never be manipulative or negative. No "you suck, you're unhealthy, you're overweight" for shock value. We're not selling anything that's damaging the world or humanity. We know every single person would be better with our service. We want to help.

—*The ability to shrug off what doesn't work and quickly move on from rejection.*

I was listening to a podcast the other day where this guy did 100 days of rejection just so he would get used to it. He'd walk up to strangers and say, "Hey can I have $100?" He'd ask businesses for free things. Or request weird random favors from people. Conclusion: Rejection is no big deal. It's going to happen. Meanwhile, he got what he wanted 51 percent of the time. Fifty-one out of 100. Imagine if we all did that with our businesses. If you try a marketing idea and it doesn't work, where's the harm?

Those are the basic guidelines, but one more thing before we dive into ideas: If I had to sum up good guerrilla marketing with one word, it would be **playfulness.**

That's the bottom line, really. Playfulness. Try one thing, mess around with another, and what about this other thing, *let's play with that.*

We have a good time doing good work, and do a good job letting everyone know about it. There are so many funny or subtle things you can do. People don't think about it, so hopefully this will get some ideas out there ...

A QUICK WORD ABOUT BUSINESS CARDS

I know a lot of people are down on business cards these days. I know younger people who think they're just not useful. Some "print" relic in a digital world. Well, if you want to be a good guerrilla marketer, you need to go back to the Stone Age, okay? Business cards are an amazing guerrilla marketing tool, perhaps one of the best.

Sure, on the surface they're nothing more than a reminder for people who sign up for or know about your service. Or a calling card. Or something a lot of people throw in the trash.

If you embrace a guerrilla mindset, however, a well-designed business card — in fact, a pocket full of them — is an invitation to play. How many creative and unexpected ways can you get your cards into people's hands so they remember you? You're going to find out soon.

34. Have a huge company logo sticker on your laptop

How many times do you find yourself working in coffee shops, hotel lobbies, airports, or anywhere other than your home or gym? When I'm working in these environments, I've found that people are curious. Not nosy, just ... checking my logo out. Right now I'm working on a new sticker that will say something like, "Ask me about personal nutrition plans" or "Visit our website." You could get a client without even talking to anyone just because you're working in a coffee shop.

35. Don't stop at your laptop

I'm having T-shirts made that say, "Ask me nutrition questions" with our logo. We already have shirts that say, "Earn your carbs." People always comment on them. They start conversations. They're clearly looking at me. And they're curious. That's your cue to go in.

Another idea: Create branded mugs for your coffee shop visits. You'll save some money and plastic, and let dozens of people a day see your logo. Maybe hundreds.

36. Encourage spontaneous Q&As in tight quarters

You know how people always tweet, "I'm waiting for a flight. AMA!" Well, do that with the folks in the airport right there with you. Tape a paper sign to your laptop

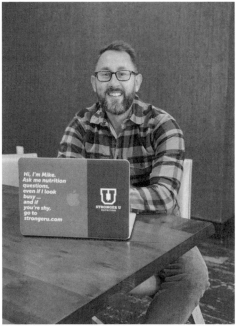

Mike in his element: sitting in a coffee shop, happy to chat with anybody who wants to know about nutrition. His computer reads "Hi, I'm Mike. Ask me nutrition questions, even if I look busy ... and if you're shy, go to strongeru.com."

that says, "We're all stuck here. Ask me anything about nutrition." Have the ancient technology known as business cards ready because the conversations will be really good.

(Also, a quick note on guerrilla idea generation. Notice how these first three kind of flow from one another? The more you think this way, the more you'll find ideas flowing like that, so be ready to capture the genius.)

37. Drop a strategic twenty, part one

Next time you buy a coffee, leave $20 with the cashier for the next few people's coffees. Tell the cashier, "If anyone asks, I'm the one who did it." Then have a seat with your laptop open (the one with the big logo and website). Someone might come over and say thank you. But at the very least, anyone who asks will get an eyeful of your logo. Pro tip: Never wear headphones or earbuds in these situations. You *want* people to approach.

38. Leave business cards in unexpected places

One of my favorite tricks is leaving my business cards in diet and nutrition books at Barnes and Noble. If the books are faced cover-out, I'll slip one between copies, too. Think about it: Anyone browsing the diet section is a warm lead. They're already looking for a healthy change.

I don't litter in public, but I leave cards all over the place. I leave cards behind in hotels, or tuck them in the drink menu when I go out to eat, or in the little wallet with the bill.

39. Double your exposure

Whenever you do some crazy stunt (like leaving cards in diet books), post it to social media. Keep it jokey and lighthearted. It enhances your rep as an interesting, playful person. A handy hashtag: #EveryDayImHustling.

40. Tape business cards to indulgent foods

I tape business cards to Halloween candy with the message, "You can eat this on our program." This works for any kind of packaged snack left out for folks.

41. Give business cards to members around major holidays

This is a big one for us at Stronger U because we really can measure the results. We'll mail a handful of business cards to clients anytime during the year when they're likely to get together with friends and family they haven't seen for a while.

The few days after Thanksgiving are our biggest sign-up days and it's not just because a bunch of people ate a lot of food and feel bad about it. It's more like: A lot of people see loved ones who work with us and are like, "Holy crap, what are you doing, you look great!" Then our clients tell them about us. How lucky, they have this antiquated technology known as a business card in their pocket.

42. Stake out your local boudoir photography studio

We have a boudoir photographer near our office (someone who takes sensual, intimate photos of folks), and the owner's clients want to look good for their shoots, so we partner up to help with that. If you don't have a local boudoir photographer (what a shame), this will work with any local business where people want to be leaner, healthier, and looking good. Some sort of a combo package offered by a wedding photographer like a "transform your body, take pictures" would be a cool upsell.

43. Send your success stories shopping

We've had a lot of clients lose weight and need new wardrobes. We'll send them gift cards to local stores (and business cards, naturally), encouraging them to shop, share their pics, and urge people to think of change. Even better: Tell them to post when they donate big bags of clothes they don't need anymore. It's a major occasion, so celebrate it. We've had people post pics of entire trash bags full of clothes.

44. Drop a strategic twenty, part two

I once put $20 in an airplane menu with a card saying, "Enjoy a meal on us. We're happy to help."

45. Join Facebook groups not related to health or fitness

Plenty of groups exist that aren't "health/wellness/ fitness"-related that have natural ties to the industry. The Instant Pot Group. Recipe groups. Groups surrounding types of foods or ways of eating. All of these people talk about food, so nutrition is bound to come up. I try to become the dude who can help with nutrition questions without selling my services. That's key: Deliver good info and stop there. Don't sell.

46. Monetize a meme

We once did a satisfaction survey that came in with *98 percent* of clients happy with us, so we created a meme and shared it. With an incentive: Everyone who shared it was eligible to win a free trip. We got more than 500 shares and had an incredibly busy two weeks after that.

47. Become a grocery store tour guide

For real. Set up a relationship with your local grocery store manager and do a free grocery store tour for people interested in eating a little healthier. Market it as a tour and Q&A to build more interest. This gives you an opportunity to teach and connect with people, and be the resource when nutrition/fitness comes up among the staff.

48. Say howdy, neighbor

Introduce yourself to your neighbors via community apps like Nextdoor. Offer Q&As, shopping trips, and training. You may become the go-to person in the area.

49. Drop a strategic twenty, part three

Next time you go through a tollbooth, use the "cash only" lane and give the attendant $20 to cover as many people behind you as possible. Some will do this, some won't. Give 'em cards for people who ask who did it. Even if the attendant pockets the cash, worst case is you lose a couple bucks and someone new knows about your brand.

50. And why not a fiver, too?

Drop a five-dollar bill on the ground with your card taped to it. At the very least, you'll make someone's day.

A final word of encouragement

I started my career in banking. They were so over-the-top, aggressive, and salesy that I had to leave the business. I just wasn't comfortable with all that pure sales stuff, all the time. One thing they'd have us do was stand outside with flyers and try to start conversations. I wasn't equipped to do that yet. I am now, mostly because of guerrilla marketing, which is an entirely different animal from what the bank did.

I don't know if people are willing to do things like that. I talk to a lot of fit pros and they want to know how we grew our business, and I ask, "If I told you to do this, this, and that, would you?" And every example I give them is some kind of guerrilla marketing I've done. And they're like "I dunno, man, that makes me uncomfortable."

Well, I'll be honest. That may be the difference between having the life you want and not having the life you want. I think about all I've done with this stuff and wonder, *What if I never did any of it?* Scary to think about.

If you took everything away from me and I had to do it all over again, I'd do the exact same things because I'm so convinced it's a proven method. No one does it. I'll be at events and people always ask, "How can I get more clients?" Someone always says, "Paid ads." I didn't do any of that. I know I speak only from my own success, but there are so many ways to get clients that people haven't even considered yet.

How do you get people to buy your stuff? Go down the rabbit hole, man.

THE TAKEAWAY

Effective guerrilla marketing requires a willingness to experiment, tapping your creativity, and the ability to quickly move on from rejection. But above all, it comes down to one word: playfulness.

PART THREE

How to Get More Referrals

CHAPTER 8

How to Create Clients Who Refer You More Clients

(and Why Most Referral Systems Are Fatally Flawed)

"A referred brand is a preferred brand; and a
preferred brand is a referred brand."
—*Bernard Kelvin Clive*
(*Ghanaian branding expert*)

Imagine the perfect prospect standing in front of you. She has specific and reachable goals and motivation to burn. Best of all, this person says in an absolutely perfect tone of voice ... "How do I buy?"

We want client conversions to be this smooth and simple, and one way to help that process is through referrals.

Referred prospects are better than cold leads in every possible way.

A referred prospect:

- converts faster
- spends more
- does much less shopping around

Referred prospects are ready to work, have increased lifetime value, and best of all, they're preconditioned to refer because that's how they were brought in.

On top of that, the customer who made the referral shows a deepened commitment to your business, improving *her* lifetime value.

This is (or should be) nothing new to you. You probably know that you should be getting referrals. So let me ask you point-blank: Do you have a system in place to generate referrals?

I'm not talking about a haphazard, "Maybe if I get the courage, I'll ask people one time and offer them a gift card if they send me somebody." That doesn't count. I'm asking whether you have an *actual systematic approach to generating referrals.*

I'm guessing no. Few do, which is a shame, because it's the single most valuable client generation strategy to have in place. After the first year, a trainer should have enough ongoing referrals feeding their business that they never have to advertise for a client again.*

Let's talk about why the most commonly used referral systems in the fitness industry are flawed, and then look at the secrets behind a much more thoughtful and effective strategy: Establishing a referral culture in and around your business.

What's a referral culture? (After reading this, you'll immediately notice what you're missing)

"Culture" refers to a social group's customs, institutions, and achievements. Not its processes or systems. That's what a referral culture looks and feels like — referrals are customary and institutionalized within your particular group (you define how large or concentrated your group is).

I've said before that some people get weird when it comes to asking for money. Same deal with referrals. Your garden-variety referral can be incredibly clumsy. A lot of times it goes like this:

> Hey, awesome client who has gotten great results.
> I, uh, have some space in my schedule and want
> to reserve it for friends and family of my awesome

---

* The exception to this, of course, is if a trainer wants to aggressively scale and grow a much bigger business. In this case, while a referral culture is still paramount to success, other forms of advertising and marketing will be necessary. But for a trainer looking to maintain a strong clientele, and even grow a company with a few other coaches, referrals are all that should be needed.

> *clients. So, um, uh, if you, uh, have somebody*
> *who wants fitness stuff and to look good and get*
> *muscle and stuff, then can you tell them to call*
> *me ... or email me? To show my appreciation*
> *to you, I'll give you a gift card, or discount on*
> *your training, or enter you in a drawing to win*
> *something.*

I exaggerate, but not much.

Don't get me wrong ... this is better than nothing. But it's flawed for a bunch of reasons:

- It's random. You have no structure to when and how you ask.

- The request doesn't take into account the psychology of why a client would *want* to refer.

- You're asking a lot and giving comparatively little. As an economic transaction, it's one-sided. The current client gets a gift card. You get a new client who could generate thousands of dollars for you.

- The client takes on a lot of risk. What if she refers a family member who has a bad experience with you? She'll hear about it at every holiday gathering for years.

- You're asking her to do something that takes her out of the natural flow of her life. Why should this busy person do something unrelated to her job or personal life for the benefit of you and your business?

Let's translate what I just showed you so you can see how it's interpreted by your client:

> *Please tell your family and friends about my training. When you do, please make sure that you accurately represent what I do, including the benefits specific to the client. If they decide to come in and give me their money, I'll give you a relatively insignificant bit of it in some form of token gesture that isn't all that meaningful to you.*

That version isn't an exaggeration at all. That's exactly what you're asking of your client. And that's exactly why so many referrals fall flat.

If somebody's going to send you business, it needs to happen when it's *natural* for her, not at the exact time you bribe her with a gift card.

Referral psychology 101

The first step? Understand why people refer, because it has little to do with any sort of external incentive. Rewards are fine as a reactionary measure of appreciation (but only if done well). Truthfully, however, they don't do much to proactively encourage referrals — which is what we're after.

A quick note before I dive in ... I readily admit that some clients will help you out of the goodness of their hearts. And, in rare cases, others will be motivated by a financial incentive. Don't depend on rare cases to grow your business, okay? Take 'em when they come, but on a bigger scale, action is primarily driven by internal motivation.

With that in mind, clients will refer if you do three things:

1. Make them feel important.
2. Help them show that they're in-the-know.
3. Make it easy for them by fitting referrals into their natural patterns.

Consider two guerrilla marketing examples from Mike in the previous chapter. First, when he gives his clients gift cards for new clothing because the old stuff doesn't fit, that's a natural way for people to go shopping and celebrate the event publicly, resulting in friends and family asking what they did to lose the weight. A similar example (that doesn't cost anything) is Mike encouraging his clients to donate their clothing that no longer fits and share the occasion publicly.

That's what I mean when I say this is a psychology lesson more than anything.

Everyone can refer. All clients of yours have relatives, friends, neighbors, coworkers, fellow church members, poker buddies, book club cohorts, and more they could recommend to your business if you make the process natural for them (and we'll talk structure and examples in the next chapter).*

If you aren't getting referrals, it's not the customer's fault. It's yours.

If you aren't getting referrals, it's not the customer's fault. It's yours.

Build your culture

Okay, so you want to establish a referral culture in your business. How do you do that? Simple: Integrate referrals into the fabric of your business, as opposed to just something you hope people will do. The easiest way to do that is to signal to everyone you work with that

---

* *Let me tell you a story about a long-term client of mine who never referred. We worked together for five years. He loved the training and was extremely well-connected and respected in the neighborhood.*

A few years in we had a conversation about why he'd never referred me a client. I don't recall how it came about. But we were close. The chat wasn't awkward.

Anyway, he told me point-blank that our sessions — Tuesdays and Thursdays at 4:30 pm — were the only times he had to himself the entire week. In order to protect that me time, he didn't want his friends coming to the same studio.

I totally got it and totally respected it. Sure, it would have been nice for him to have sent me other clients, but he knew I didn't really need it. By that time, I was already referring my overload of clients to other trainers (and making additional commissions for it). That, and this client spent tens of thousands on training with me over the years. I was happy for him to have the space and time he needed.

So, while every client can refer, not every client will refer. And that's fine.

referrals "are what we do here," as opposed to conveying something like, "referrals are appreciated."

Your referral culture statement and expectations should be part of your onboarding process. Your "this is what we do here" declaration. Keep in mind that you don't want to make it sound like marching orders. Always be friendly. This is just another part of your story, but something you value and encourage.

Author and entrepreneur Dan Kennedy developed a list that helps define referral culture to clients. This is not something you would publish. Instead, use the following as a guide, attempting to ingrain all points into your business over time. Here's Kennedy's list with a few slight adaptations from me to make it specific to fit pros:

1. Our customers refer.
2. Our good customers refer often.
3. Our best customers refer often and a lot.
4. Referrals are expected. From you.
5. Referrals are genuinely appreciated.
6. People you refer will be well taken care of. You'll only get happy reports and thanks from those you refer.
7. Not referring is weird. If for any reason you don't feel comfortable referring us to someone, please let us know how we can do better. Because we will.
8. There are lots of different reasons people do business with us — not just the reason that brought you in. Keep all of these reasons in mind.

9. Most people don't really know how to find a good, trustworthy fitness professional, so you're doing others a great service by telling them about us.
10. There are easy ways to introduce people to us and get our information into the hands of people you think we can be of service to.
11. Here's how: (provide exact steps).

People do all sorts of things for emotional self-interest, even though they may consciously think (and would certainly insist) they're doing these things "for" someone out of love, appreciation, friendship, charity, or generosity. If there's one uniting motivation affecting everybody, every single day, it's pursuit of feeling good about themselves and how they feel they're being viewed by others.

If you take this into account and request your referrals in a way that's natural for your client, and as you've seen here, welcome all clients into your warm and friendly referral culture, you'll be swimming in high-quality leads.

What if someone says, "I can't refer you because X"?

Nobody's perfect. And it's entirely possible a client won't feel comfortable referring you because of some reason you may not even be aware of. I don't mean someone acting on a weird personal principle like Mr. Pink in *Reservoir Dogs* ("I don't tip"). I'm talking about reasons related to your service excellence, or lack thereof.

If you've truly established a referral culture, all your clients know how important referrals are to you. If someone for some reason won't refer you, *it's a big deal.* You need to know what's going on, and now, because you also need to prevent the client's *anti*-referral from going out (there is such a thing as bad publicity in the fitness industry).

Mark Fisher at Mark Fisher Fitness uses a Net Promoter Score, a tool for identifying issues clients may have with his team's service. Aside from communicating well and asking clients for feedback during training (which all fit pros should be doing), Mark also sends his clients an automated email whenever they finish a program.

It asks one question: "On a scale of one to 10, how likely are you to refer us?"

The number is that client's Net Promoter Score. And the team's reaction to it is just as simple as the question itself.

- Anything below eight and the team immediately follows up with the client about how to do better.
- Nine and 10 scores generate an automated follow-up giving the client a bunch of ways to refer.

You can't lose with a system like this. Either you have happy clients referring people to you, or you find out exactly what went wrong along the way and fix the problem.

And yeah, that's the unspoken thing in a referral culture

I shouldn't have to spell out here, but I will. Referrals are all about excellence. You'll have zero credibility declaring your "referral culture" if you're constantly giving clients reasons not to refer you.

Let's move on now to the next chapter where you'll learn some specific referral strategies that put into practice the lessons you just learned.

THE TAKEAWAY

A referral culture isn't just occasionally asking clients to refer you. It's letting them know they've joined a warm and friendly environment where referrals are simply what everyone does. Referrals are expected, and if a client can't give one, follow up on the reasons and fix the problem.

CHAPTER 9

Guaranteed Systems, Strategies, and Scripts for Generating Referrals

"One customer, well taken care of, could be more valuable than $10,000 worth of advertising."

—Jim Rohn

Now that you understand the difference between a referral culture and just asking for the occasional good word, you need to bring that culture to life as a functioning system. It must be as effortless as possible for you and your clients.

The interesting part? We're not talking about a one-size-fits-all proposition. Referral systems can take forms as limitless as your imagination, as long as they work. This chapter will lay out some specific examples. They're effective, but you don't have to use them. It's more important for you to understand what those examples accomplish.

Again, your referral culture is part of your business culture and any system you implement should reflect you. Now, I get it — that sentence suggests a long, thorough thought process about how to develop your referral system. That's up to you. But super-simple works, too. That's why the examples in this chapter will vary in their complexity. What do they have in common? They're guaranteed to work.

Let's start with simple ...

The most basic referral script ever

The longer you work in this business, the more you see how getting all the referrals you need is both an art and a science. You'll get better as you go. Your approach will evolve, too. But a referral stripped down to its essence is asking a favor. While this doesn't represent a well-thought-out referral culture, it's a good start and you can employ it right away.

First things first: Don't be shy. And don't worry about hurting your existing relationship with your clients — for the most part, they want to support you.

They may have no idea how your business works and how crucial referrals are to your success. So tell them (hopefully the info from last chapter has you planning how to do this already). If they know your success is dependent on referrals, they'll be more open to sending you one.

So how do you ask? Here's the most basic script ever.

At the end of a session, either during a stretch or as the client preps to leave, say, "Thanks again for your great work today. You really smashed those deadlifts. There's something I'd love to have a quick chat with you about if that's all right." Make the compliment specific and ask if it's all right to keep him a moment longer.

"I've noticed that I'm going to have some gaps in my schedule coming up due to some personal issues with a couple of other clients, so I'm asking my existing clients first if they know anybody who might be interested in training. I want to make sure I keep the spots open to look after my clients' friends and family first before marketing to the outside world. Do you know anybody who might be interested?"

At this point your client will hopefully mention someone. If he doesn't, no problem. Thank him for his time and say goodbye. You can follow up next time. If the client has suggested someone, ask if the person has any specific fitness goals or issues. If he says something like, "Well, he hurt his shoulder recently," you can respond, "You know, I have a lot of experience working with shoulder injuries and am happy to reach out to get the details. Do you mind asking him for permission for me to call?"

The client will almost always say yes, and then never follow up.

Your client is busy and he'll forget to pass along your info, or won't bother, or will feel awkward about the entire thing because it's unnatural for him. This isn't a dig on your client. Making your referral takes time. Don't make it awkward by asking him repeatedly. Instead, follow up.

Without telling him you're going to send it, find a great article on whatever condition his friend has and how to rehab it. You get double points if you wrote it yourself. Send it to your client, asking him to pass it along to his friend later that night or the next day.

The material adds value to your services and provides a non-intrusive nudge to your client to pass along the info. It also gives your client an easy segue to talk about you.

Once your client does pass on the info, he will surely preface it with, "My trainer asked me to pass this on to you," or better yet, "my awesome/stupendous/butt-kicking supertrainer asked me to pass this on to you." Make sure your email signature includes your contact info at the bottom and, once your client comes in to the gym next, if it hasn't happened already, ask for contact info to give his friend a call.

Again, that's a very simple and effective script, but

it doesn't totally eliminate the problem of making a referral part of the natural flow of a client's life. That could be the biggest challenge for you. Let's look at some other examples.

HOW TO REWARD REFERRALS

It's become common practice to reward a referral with a free session or something similar. This is a terrible referral incentive. It's not memorable, personal, or special in any way. Your client has already accepted paying for sessions.

Instead, I recommend offering a "gift worth up to $X" (the amount being whatever you want to give). When a client sends you a new prospect, take the opportunity to show you care about him on a personal level. The most meaningful gestures are not the most expensive, they're the ones that are the most gratuitous. Taking a little effort to do or get something you know is special to him is way more impactful than buying a gift card.

Use this opportunity to strengthen the relationship. If she loves the opera, get her tickets. If he's a huge football fan, get him a jersey of his favorite player (vintage jerseys are particularly awesome for die-hard fans). Over the course of your training, gather intel into what your client deeply cares about. Then wait for opportunities

> *like referrals to show how much you were*
> *listening and how you care. Paying attention to*
> *those little things goes a long way.*

Every client gets a referral card on day one

Real estate marketing expert Craig Proctor has a brilliant referral system, and I've made some adjustments to it relevant to the fitness industry. Basically, the referral process begins the day you sign a new client.

Three things need to happen as soon as a client signs:

1. Thank them for their business.
2. Give them a sense of the next steps.
3. Ask them for referrals and equip them with a tool that makes it easy.

The "make it easy" part is the challenge. In Proctor's example, he gives his new customers printed, postage-paid referral cards. Each card includes all the pertinent information about the business. All the client has to do is fill in a few lines and drop it in a mailbox.

One key feature of the card is what Proctor calls WIFM (what's in it for me?). By promising a donation to a worthy local charity in return for a referral, the new client feels good about sending business your way.

To make it work, you need to say the right things when offering the card. Here's a script:

"Thanks for putting your health in our hands. I can't wait to help you achieve (client's goal here). Now that we have the paperwork signed, here's precisely what's going to happen next (lay out the next steps). If you have any questions about the steps, I'm happy to address them.

"In my experience, when people start this process, they develop a heightened awareness of others looking to begin their own fitness journey. If you come across someone who shows interest in starting a fitness program, I'd appreciate it if you pass along my card, and then fill out this referral card and drop it in the mail to me. (Hand over both cards.)

"I'm asking you to do this not out of self-interest, but to help those in need. When you refer somebody who begins with us, I donate a portion of the revenue to (name of local charity). So in addition to assuring the best possible service and results for your friend or coworker, you'll also be supporting (the charity)."

Here's what the card will look like:

Your Referrals Help [CHARITY]

Help us help {Children, homeless, disabled, etc.}. Our fitness company believes in giving back. When you refer a friend or family member to us who is considering starting a fitness program, you're also helping {insert charity name} achieve {insert charity goal}.

It's easy to refer your friend or family member considering starting a fitness program. Simply complete the information below and drop this card in the nearest mailbox.

Your name
_____

Their name
_____

_____   _____
Their phone #   Their email

Your Referrals Help [CHARITY]

INFORMATION ABOUT THE CHARITY

INSERT your
mailing address here

Put it in a letter

Another way to ask for referrals is not to ask for referrals. Wait, what? Instead of putting the bite on a customer to refer somebody, you're going to write a letter to new prospects. The catch: This letter will be from one of your happy clients. Think of it as a promotional piece. The happy client can write it, or you can write it and they'll edit and sign off on it.

The letter will describe the client's initial skepticism

and how her life has been changed because of the transformation. If your client is okay with it, include before-and-after pictures. Then, at the end, include a special offer for "friends of (your client)." A gift card or complimentary week of sessions works well.

The better you paint a picture of her beginning state, skepticism, and ultimate transformation, the better the letter will perform. The beauty of it: Once written, you have a go-to referral tool easily deployed for months or even years. Mail to the neighborhood surrounding your gym, prospects, stale leads, and anybody else.

It may also be helpful, if your client is willing, to include the client's contact information in case the prospect has any questions. Then provide your client with a script on how to respond to these questions. Don't leave anything to chance. (Some clients may not want to go this far. That's okay. The letter by itself will be powerful.)

If your client likes to write, he or she can compose a letter. Better though is to provide a questionnaire and then you write the letter (or you hire a writer to do it).

Here's a sample questionnaire:

1. Why did you join the gym?
2. What were your past experiences with gyms and trainers?
3. Why did you decide to train with me?
4. What were your goals when you began training?
5. What are your goals now?

6. Have your family and friends been supportive? If so, how? If not, how?
7. Have there been any negatives during this journey?
8. What would you say to somebody considering joining the gym?

One or two great letters will perform better than any marketing flyer you could imagine. To show you what I mean, here's part of an actual letter written by one of my clients years ago. Names have been changed, but the letter is real. Read it and you'll immediately see the power in it. To be blunt, this is the best piece of promotional material I have ever seen produced for the fitness industry. You could fill a gym with a letter like this.

TALES FROM THE GYM FLOOR: HOW I JOINED THE GYM AND FOUND RELIGYM!

Joining the gym was the single best thing I have done for myself in the last year. I have had a few failed gym experiences in the past. I'm not sure why I felt compelled to make another attempt at something which was probably not going to work. There were definite reasons that I felt compelled to try something.

1. HEALTH: My doctor was threatening to put me on drugs to control an increasing cholesterol rate. Heart problems, stroke, and diabetes have struck pretty much every blood relative of mine and I knew that these were going to be my problems if I didn't do something to prevent that from happening.

2. AGE/VANITY: I joined the gym about 3 weeks after my 49th (ew, yuck) birthday. I still don't feel that old! I couldn't believe what birthday was going to happen to me next. Even more, I hated thinking of myself as being old, fat, and ugly. I teach in a school where the majority of teachers are in their 20s, some in their 30s. Being so terribly out of shape made me feel very inferior — and I am just not inferior! Many people seem to regard overweight people as lacking self-control, as being stupid or uninteresting. Those are not my negative qualities (I do have lots of other ones), but I felt that people did not really see my strengths because they did not look deeper than the exterior.

3. STRESS: My husband has had cancer for many years. He's had numerous operations which have taken a severe toll on his lifestyle, and therefore, the lives of my children and me. The past two years have been impossible; heavy doses of chemo and steroids have altered his intellect and personality. The cancer and treatments have led to other health problems. It's very lonely to

*live with someone whose main focus in life is his
own survival. It's tiring to be the only capable
parent in a household. It's depressing to watch
someone slowly, slowly die.*

*Even worse was finding out that my spouse's
cancer was caused by a gene which he may have
passed on to my children. Adding all of this to
everyday stress was almost unbearable. For the
first time in my entire life, I was really frightened
by depression. This was such a dramatic contrast
to my usual personality — optimistic, happy,
cheerful. I am not a quitter. I knew that I had
to take charge of my situation. While I could
not change all of my problems, I could change
some of them and put up a good fight against the
others. That's why I decided to try the gym one
more time.*

Gym memberships

*I joined Body and Soul gym in December, 2009.
Previously I belonged to:*

*The gym at Yorkdale shopping mall (don't
remember the name) many years ago — huge
disaster. Way too busy.*

*The Dunfield Club — because that was the gym
of my trainer/friend at the time. It was nice, but*

too big and impersonal. I don't remember why I stopped going.

A women-only gym at Bayview and Eglinton (about 10 years ago). It was okay, but I had no positive results and just stopped going.

Body and Soul when it first opened. I enjoyed it for about 3 or 4 months. The membership had started with a physical assessment. I had a reassessment after 3 or 4 months which showed very little improvement! That was very discouraging. I kept my membership for another 6 months, but this was during a particularly stressful period with my husband's illness. For the final 3 months of the membership, I did not enter the gym once.

Trainers over the years

I worked with 4 trainers before working with Jonathan Goodman.

The first was a friend who was just getting into the business. She was pretty tough and I saw good results. I enjoyed working with her. I don't remember why we stopped.

The second trainer was through a package offered at the women's gym. I worked with the trainer the gym suggested, though I would not have chosen her myself. I didn't really like her as a person; she was not too bright and had no personality. I could not wait for the prepaid sessions to end and did not see any results. I had the impression that gyms pushed trainers in order to make extra money off the clients (yes, I really thought that!).

The third trainer was (name omitted) at Body and Soul. She was great! We had a lot of fun together. I felt that I was working hard and having fun but, as I mentioned above, did not really get any visible results from the sessions. I got tired of working with her even though I really liked her as a person. I canceled a number of sessions and was always pleased when she had to cancel an appointment. We worked together twice a week, every week, which, in retrospect, may have been too often. I work well by myself.

The fourth trainer was (name omitted) at Body and Soul. When I rejoined Body and Soul last December, he approached me regarding training sessions. At that point, I thought it would be a good idea to work with someone to get started with a proper gym plan. Things went well at first, but I soon realized that he was not the right person for me. He was often not available for sessions, so I would be repeating the same things too many times. He sometimes did not follow through with answers to questions, or the answers did not sound right. Coincidentally, he left the gym at that point, just as I was wondering how to tactfully negotiate a change of trainer. I was already pretty sure that I wanted to work with Jon.

So, finally, here is the good part of my story. ***With all those past gym experiences that did not work out or were not so memorable, why is my current gym experience working so well?***

I really like my gym. It is close to home, which is really important. I usually go to the gym before going home from work so that I don't get distracted, which might prevent me from doing a workout. While I don't really know the other clients at the gym, I think they are probably pretty much from my neighborhood, so there is a familiar feel about them.

I like the size of the gym — small and personal, yet not so small that I have to wait for machines or work too closely next to someone I don't know. I like the aesthetic of the gym — simple white walls and open beamed ceilings. One of the trainers once mentioned to me in passing that Body and Soul is a "nerdy" gym — I find that thought appealing!

*I have had more than a few conversations
with various trainers about books, opera, and
Beethoven — that was unexpected! The people
who work at the gym are all incredibly nice.
In my first months at the gym, I was so self-
conscious that I found it hard to even say hello to
them. Now pretty much everyone talks to me —
which I love.*

*One of the trainers gives me little health insights,
one chats with me about music and concerts,
and another often compliments me on my
progress. It is very welcoming to work out in this
environment; it makes me more comfortable. It's
a bit disappointing on days when the trainers are
not in because it feels more impersonal.*

How did I choose my trainer / how did I know he was the right one?

*As I think he knows, I really attribute the positive
results to Jon. I have worked with lots of people
one-on-one in a music setting (very similar to the
trainer/client experience) and I know that the
teacher/student relationship has to be just right
for everything to work.*

When I was still training with (name omitted),

I would watch Jon work with clients; he seemed tough, but also lots of fun. This is exactly the way I teach and I thought Jon would be a good match for me. Having gotten to know him better, I also find him very intelligent, ambitious, courteous, thoughtful, and insightful — all qualities that I admire and need from someone to whom I look for advice.

I learned a long time ago that if I could walk all over somebody, I inevitably would. I think that's why I wrote off the other trainers. Jon seemed far more formidable than that! In our initial sessions, I was scared that, if I wasn't good enough, he would give me the boot. That fear must have come from my music-student experience, because I no longer have that impression; however, it got me off to a diligent start. Now I enjoy working with Jon because I see the great progress I have made, in strength, overall fitness and weight loss. I enjoy working with Jon because I respect him. Whenever I have a question or want to schedule some sessions, he often responds to my emails within minutes. I really appreciate that.

In the months we have been working together, I have not had any injuries — that's fantastic! I really trust that he is having me do things I am capable of, while still pushing forward to tougher things. I enjoy all the positive reinforcement, but I also appreciate that he made me work pretty hard for about 2 months before he coughed up a solid compliment. I think that Jon is an amazing teacher. When I have trouble picking up something new, he is good at breaking it down into smaller steps.

It seems that I have made all this progress in a seamless fashion. In retrospect, I don't have the impression that I've been working hard; I just feel like I've been having fun. I really like Jon as a person, and I think he really understands what makes me tick. I am certain that this is why things have gone so well. With other trainers, I always reached a point where I just wanted the sessions to stop so that I could do my own thing. With Jon, that hasn't happened once. I look forward to every session and can't wait to see what is coming next. I am also pretty impressed that he asked me to write this letter — I'm glad that he is interested in my opinion!

Nutrition

It is pretty much an accepted fact that, in order to lose weight, you need to combine exercise with proper diet. It was very convenient that Jon could help me with both. In the past months, I have *totally changed the way I eat. What I liked the most about the way he changed my diet was that he changed things in small steps.*

Jon didn't try to do a sudden overhaul of my diet — just made little suggestions that were easy to gradually fit in with what I was already doing. Initially, it was very helpful to submit the daily eating sheets. I really did not want to hand in a sheet filled with embarrassing (stupid) food choices, so it made me really think more carefully about what I was eating. It was very helpful that he didn't mind me handing him those sheets for about 2 months!

I have reached a point where I really have control over what I am eating. *I can walk into Phipps and buy a bagful of goodies for someone else without buying a single treat for myself. I can walk past a plateful of cookies sitting on a table without even wanting to eat one. I still use the nutrition sheets sometimes when I start to get off track. There have been days when my entire carb/produce intake was a banana and a glass of wine.*

Past goals

When I rejoined the gym last December, I set 2 easy goals for myself:

1. *to get to the gym a minimum of twice a week*

2. *to try to get my weight at least below 150*
   (from a starting point of 173 — oy)

I find this so hard to imagine now, that the first time back on the treadmill last December, I was actually shaking. I was under so much stress at the time that I can still remember that moment. There is certainly something therapeutic about hiding behind the headphones and just pounding away on a treadmill for 45 minutes. I think that is why it was easy to get to the gym regularly in those first weeks.

Being at the gym is all about me. No one asks me to do anything for them at the gym. This is partially why I now go to the gym every day — it is my moment for myself, which rarely happens at home or at work. Also, by going every single day, I never think about which days I should go and which ones to take off. I just always go, like always brushing my teeth. That way I never worry about missing a day here or there.

It took about 9 months to lose 25 pounds. I didn't think it would take that long. This has definitely been the hardest part of my story. I know that it is somewhat irrelevant. In spite of the number on the scale, I know that I look and feel a lot better today than I did one year ago.

Future goals

1. *I still think that I should probably weigh about 10 or 20 pounds less than I do, but this is not my main focus anymore.*

2. *I want to be sure to maintain at least a 5-day-a-week gym habit (and preferably stick to the 7-day plan) and not lose any ground on my eating habits. I still need to eat more raw vegetables and fruit.*

3. *This past summer I spent an incredibly happy week in Cape Breton. While the trip was full of great and varied experiences, I truly loved getting exercise in natural surroundings — hiking and kayaking. These are things I NEVER do at home and haven't done in such a long time.*

Support / reactions from friends and family

Fortunately, I have not had much negative response to this lifestyle change. My husband does not like the change of cuisine — he needs more carbs and less protein in his diet, which is the opposite of what I need. He cooks a lot more for himself now. My daughter complains frequently

*that I get home later from work and so spend
less time with her. I'm glad that my teenager still
wants to spend time with me.*

*Many of my friends make regular comments
on my new and improved look. Some people
have never commented — I don't know if this is
passive negativity or just a polite reluctance to
acknowledge that I used to look not so great. I
recently forwarded a Body and Soul promotion to
several friends — there was not one taker. That's
a shame.* **More people need to know about
this place.**

Negatives

*There are definitely negatives to the intense gym
experience. Expenditure of time and money
are the obvious big issues. Additionally though,
when I get home at 6:30 after a full day of
work plus a serious workout, I am often really
tired. I don't feel like cooking or emptying the
dishwasher. My house has never looked worse. I
am procrastinating on a lot of small things. I'm
getting too accustomed to compliments — it's
time to get over that.*

*I also worry that maybe I am getting a bit too
independent and self-focused. With the same
control that lets me walk by a plate of cookies*

without even wanting to have one, I have managed to completely shut out my husband's medical issues from my emotions — which is a lot healthier for me but maybe not so nice.

I am worried that I will, at some point, fall back to old habits, stop coming to the gym, start eating too much, regain weight. This is why I am afraid to eat even 1 cookie or miss 1 day of going to the gym. I don't know what would happen if my gym would close. I am very connected to this place — I find it hard to think of going anywhere else. Additionally, I am worried that Jon is going to move along at some point, and my good luck story will end. I have connected so much of my progress to the fact that he works so well for me.

Emotions

I find it interesting that, in Jon's written request for this story, he asked for "brutal honesty" and descriptions of emotion. I did not anticipate any emotional connection with a gym. On the surface, going to the gym should be as simple as pushing weights up and down, over and over again.

Over the past 3 or 4 months, people have told me almost daily that I look great, fantastic. That has had a huge impact on my sense of well-being. For me to spend one to two hours EVERY DAY on MYSELF rather than on my family has had a tremendous impact on my sense of independence.

This past summer, planning a trip by myself and for myself when my family was trying so hard to get me to do the group thing with them — I felt that was a big deal for me. I would not have done it a year ago. That summer trip gave me back my "happy place." I remember doing an exercise with Jon one day; he told me to think of my happy place, and all I could think was "how pathetic, I don't have one."

My life is going to change completely in the next two or three years as my children leave home, and I will probably no longer have a husband. Change can be good, but also stressful ... strength is crucial for me as I feel this looming. A simple thing like being able to jump four step boxes is symbolic of conquering fear and having power and control. It also brings me back to my happy place — on a mountain, in a forest, beside the water, leaping over logs. Imagine!

Conclusions

- It never hurts to try just one more time.

- My gym is comfortable and has a unique personality. Some people hate going to the *gym — I love going to mine. It's good to actually find a place you enjoy visiting every day.*

- *Start slowly with small expectations and then build up.*

- *I was so intimidated in the gym at first and felt sort of out-of-place. I didn't talk to anyone unless they spoke to me first. Do other people feel that way at first?*

- *To choose a trainer, spend a few hours on the treadmill analyzing the people on the gym floor. Figure out whose style might match your personality. Don't just sign on with the person who asks you or a new trainer the gym is trying to push.*

- *Keep a training journal to track progress. I didn't, but wish I had. Writing this has been enlightening. It is very encouraging to look back over the past months, think about the what, why, and how, and to realize what a positive force the gym has been for me.*

Happy tales from the gym floor

One day when my son (name omitted) was at The Running Room, talking about all the stuff he was up to, he was asked if anyone else in his

family was athletic. He told them, "My mom is."
That made me happy!

One day my friend Sue went home from work
and was telling her husband about something
I had said. He asked her, "Who is Elizabeth?"
She replied, "You know, we sat with her at
Melissa's wedding ... brown hair, red dress, she
has the daughter graduating from Harvard."
His response — "How can she have a daughter
graduating from Harvard? She's like 35 years
old." Please refer back to the 2nd reason I joined
the gym ... YAY YAY YAY!!!

This summer I went hiking with 2 teenage
athletes and a triathlete and it was ME who led
the pace ... and I wasn't even pushing all that
hard!

I can get my heart rate up to 186. Please refer
back to the 1st reason that I joined the gym!

Last September, for the beginning of the school
year, I was buying pants in size 12. This year,
the new clothes were either size 6 or 4. That's a
miracle.

One day, during a session with Jon, one of his
clients asked him a question, after which he
turned to me and made a comment about how

well I have been doing and that I could be the poster girl for the gym! Ha ha ha. I was mildly embarrassed, but I sure told lots of friends about that. I love compliments.

At the gym today, I bench-pressed 95 pounds and deadlifted 125 pounds. I love telling people that. And that's just today.

When I joined the gym last December, I was a wreck. Today, I am once again the person I have always thought myself to be — strong and happy, bouncing off the walls. I accomplished that by myself with a lot of help from Jon.

Our business deals with real people living real lives and we can have a massive positive impact on everybody we train. Your referral asks, no matter how you decide to format them, are the ideal time to showcase the best of this positivity.

THE TAKEAWAY

Your referral system cannot be haphazard. It can evolve over time as you get better at asking for referrals, but find a method you like that gets results. Experiment. Refine. Always emphasize your care for your clients and be genuine.

AFTERWORD

You'll Figure It Out

In order to develop tremendous confidence in your own abilities, you must have courage.

Courage to ideate and courage to create.

Nobody is born with courage. It develops when things don't go your way. Courage develops when you fail.

You cannot fail if you don't try — so try a lot and fail a lot. So long as your failures are not catastrophic, embrace them. The punishment for failure is never as bad as we fear it will be. Acknowledgement of this forms courage.

In most cases, failing is not absolute. Instead, it represents a new challenge — one you didn't account for — one that forces you to figure out a solution.

And, over time, you become pretty good at figuring it out. And, over some more time, you get pretty confident that no matter what happens, you'll figure it out.

None of this happens if you don't try stuff. So try stuff. You'll figure it out.

HUNGRY FOR MORE?

Catapult your training career and business today!

*Get Jonathan Goodman's other books directly at our store at **theptdc.com/store***

or worldwide on Amazon

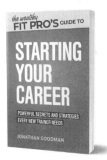

The Wealthy Fit Pro's Guide to
Starting Your Career

WWW.THEPTDC.COM/STORE

Navigate the stages of your career from certification to landing a job to continuing education. This book also talks about getting clients, building programs, and, of course, developing multiple income streams.

AVAILABLE IN*:

- PAPERBACK
- KINDLE
- AUDIBLE

*Free audio and digital with every paperback purchase

"Jon Goodman is the ultimate resource for everything regarding starting, maintaining and flourishing a fitness business. Any trainer worth their salt has at least one of his books."

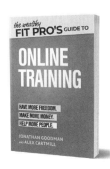

The Wealthy Fit Pro's Guide to
Online Training

WWW.THEPTDC.COM/STORE

Online fitness training is the gateway for trainers and gym owners to make more in less time with a better schedule while helping more people.

Ambitious fitness pros can now train clients from anywhere in the world if they have the knowledge and drive to do the job right — and this book will show the way.

AVAILABLE IN*:

- PAPERBACK
- KINDLE
- AUDIBLE

*Free audio and digital with every paperback purchase

"You won't find a more authoritative or comprehensive resource on the biggest opportunity for fitness professionals."

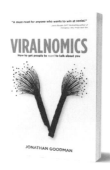

Viralnomics:
How to Get People to *Want* to Talk About You

WWW.THEPTDC.COM/STORE

Growing the PTDC to the largest independent community of personal trainers in the world was no accident. In *Viralnomics* Jon finally shares the strategies for growing a platform online while developing a fantastic audience. Oh yeah, and there's cartoons.

AVAILABLE IN:

📖 PAPERBACK

⬜ KINDLE

🔊 AUDIBLE

"A must-read for anyone who wants to win at social."

– Jonah Berger

NYT bestselling author of Contagious: Why Things Catch On

Personal Trainer Pocket Book:
A Handy Reference for All Your Daily Questions

WWW.THEPTDC.COM/STORE

From the UK to Canada, United States to Australia, and everywhere in between, Jonathan Goodman has been answering questions about succeeding in personal training to 100's of thousands of trainers worldwide since 2009. For the first time ever, these 48 answers have all been compiled into one handy reference — no stone is left unturned in this invaluable resource.

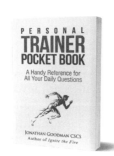

AVAILABLE IN:

📖 PAPERBACK

⬜ KINDLE

"Finally, a guide that answers all of your questions about personal training!"

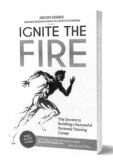

Ignite the Fire

WWW.THEPTDC.COM/STORE

Repeatedly called one of the "best books for personal trainers," *Ignite* provides a clear road map to growing your personal training career. From getting your certification to taking care of your clients, you'll learn the best, high-integrity techniques to get more clients, run a fitness business, and have a solid system for selling personal training.

AVAILABLE IN:

📕 PAPERBACK

▢ KINDLE

🔊 AUDIBLE

"A look at personal training that goes beyond the textbooks."

– Muscle & Fitness Magazine

The Highly Wealthy Online Trainer Box Set

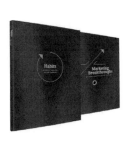

WWW.THEPTDC.COM/STORE

In this two-book limited edition box set you are about to learn both the habits needed to BREAK FREE and the marketing breakthroughs essential to CREATING BUZZ around your services.

AVAILABLE IN:

📕 PAPERBACK

"Jonathan Goodman has been responsible for helping more fitness professionals gain wealth with online training than anybody else I know."

– Dr. John Berardi

Build an Online Fitness Business

WE GUARANTEE IT

The Online Trainer Academy Certification and Mentorship is designed to get fit pros, gym owners, and nutrition coaches predictable results by adding an online fitness component to their services. If you're ready to help more people, make more money, and have more freedom, then OTA is for you.

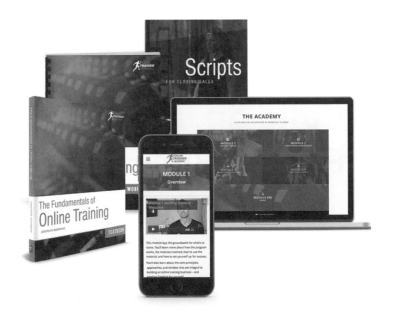

Also by Jonathan Goodman and the Personal Trainer Development Center

Books

The Wealthy Fit Pro's Guides
Starting Your Career (Book 1)
Online Training (Book 2)
Getting Clients and Referrals (Book 3)

Ignite the Fire: The Secrets to Building a Successful Personal Training Career (Revised, Updated, and Expanded)

Personal Trainer Pocket Book: A Handy Reference for All Your Daily Questions

Viralnomics: How to Get People to <u>Want</u> to Talk About You

The Highly Wealthy Online Trainer box set:
Habits of Highly Wealthy Online Trainers (Book 1)
Marketing Breakthroughs of Highly Wealthy Online Trainers (Book 2)

All titles and an updated book list available at **theptdc.com/store.**

Children's Book

Adventure, Adventure Awaits for Us All
with Alison Goodman
Available on Amazon

Courses & Certifications

Online Trainer Academy
A comprehensive certification in online training
theptdc.com/ota

Advanced Marketing Resource

Fitness Marketing Monthly — The Complete Collection
theptdc.com/fmm